How Long Will This Take? I Have Stuff to Do.

Real Stories from a Small-Town ER

Kerry Hamm

Disclaimer:
Names, locations, and portions of the details
included in this book have been altered to
protect the privacy of those involved

Just in case you haven't read my first book, let me fill you in.

With six trauma bays, one mental health room, one low pressure room, one quarantine room, and 11 other exam bays, this ER has the capacity to fit 21 patients at a time, with more than 100 patients often lining up in the lobby and waiting room on any given evening shift.

We're no big-shot inner city hospital. We transfer out burns and severe pediatric cases. We have a mental health floor, inpatient rehab, intermediate care/critical care, and hospice floor in addition to pediatrics, general surgery, obstetrics, and nursery floors. Unless patients are directly admitted from facilities in surrounding areas, they show up in our department first. Typically, we don't see many gunshot wounds or stabbings, but what does come through the doors keeps us all on our toes.

My name is Kerry and I'm the first person you'll see when you come through those ER doors: registration. Two to three clerks work during the day and evening shifts, taking turns gathering names, birth dates, and diagnoses at the front (while juggling floor transfers, admits from surrounding hospitals, and outside phone calls from some cat lady named Linda who's making her third call this shift to see if we think she needs to come in for tingling in her left butt cheek), and then in the back, where we enter patients' rooms to gather contact and insurance information to complete the registration process. Once 11 p.m. hits, I wave to my coworkers as they walk out the door, and I'm left at the registration desk with a triage nurse in a small room behind the desk, security lurking behind a two-way mirror that takes up an entire wall in front of the registration desk, a not-so-empty waiting room to my right, and six registered nurses and one or two doctors in the back.

My first book was filled with silly things patients brought to nurses and doctors. This one...eh...things get nasty—like downright *disgusting* at times. But it's all part of the job, right?

In these true stories, dialogue has been changed slightly, all names have been changed, and some situations have been slightly altered to protect patient privacy.

When Pigs Fly (You're in Bigger Trouble)

When a cop car pulled up on a Sunday overnight shift, I can't say I was the least bit surprised. Although the purchase of alcohol is banned on Sundays in this area, the ER sees the most ETOH patients and those brought in by police officers for lab work or medical clearance on this night than any other.

While I expected the patient to be intoxicated, I didn't expect the rest.

My eyes darted from side to side when the officer walked him in. The patient was in his early 30s, I think, and he was bleeding from a rather nasty wound on his arm.

He was also covered from head to toe in mud and feces and left a trail of both as he approached the desk.

"Uh," I started, so lost in trying to imagine what happened that I couldn't form a sentence.

"Medical clearance," the cop said with a smile.

I nodded and took the patient's information.

"Okay," I finally announced, "I just *have* to know what happened to you tonight."

The patient grumbled and rolled his eyes.

The officer ribbed the man. "Go on, tell her what you did to be in here tonight."

"I fell," the patient muttered. I could hardly hear him.

"You *fell?*" asked the cop. "Now, is that *all?* What'd you fall in?"

The patient shifted his weight.

"Mud."

"Just mud?"

No, not just mud. I could *smell* it.

"Probably a little bit of hog crap, too."

"Yeah," I commented, "probably just a little bit."

The cop was getting a kick out of this. "Now what were you doing, exactly, when you managed to get yourself covered in this mess?"

Our patient hesitated and finally said in a low groan, "Antagonizing the hogs."

"Antagonizing the hogs, ladies and gentlemen," the officer announced to the empty lobby. He looked back to the patient. "And how'd that work out for you?"

The mud-covered patient sniffled and looked away. "Hog bit me."

"Took a pretty good chunk out of his arm, too," the officer told me.

"Was it your hog?" I stupidly asked.

"Nope," the patient replied.

The rest of story was told by the cop.

Our patient, I guess, decided to throw a few

back and go for a drive on the back roads. He passed a pig farm and decided it would be a good idea to jump in one of the pens and scare the animals by chasing them. He fell a few times, but never one to give up, he just picked himself up and kept going. When he became bored with one fenced section, he hopped to the next, where a mother was feeding her newborn piglets. She didn't take so kindly to a drunk madman near her offspring and charged at the man. He tried to run, but fell again, and when he did, mom bit down hard on the man's forearm. His screams woke the owner of the pig farm-an elderly man across the road-and the police were called.

The patient received a few stitches for his arm and was carted off to jail.

In all the times I've drank, I can proudly say I've never been charged or bitten by a pig, brought to the hospital to be sewn up, and then taken to the slammer covered in poop. But at least that patient had an interesting story to tell when he was sober again.

Inquiring Minds Want to Know

A female patient approached the desk and stated she needed to be seen because she 'wasn't sure' how many tampons she had inside of her.

My male coworker stayed quiet throughout the registration process and did a pretty good job of keeping a straight face.

"I think I put in one without taking the first one out," the patient told me. "Now I don't feel well at all."

I nodded and told her the triage nurse would call her name soon.

As soon as the nurse finished the triage process and guided the patient around the corner, my coworker spun around in his chair like he'd been dying to keep a secret for 18 years.

"Okay," he said, "I just have to know. Is this a real thing? Does this really happen?"

I shrugged. "I guess so."

He gasped. "No way. So, like, you and all your friends and stuff, you guys have to worry about this?"

"Well," I started, hoping to explain.

"I'm so glad I'm not a woman," he replied with a sigh of relief.

I didn't try to explain anything to him. According to the patient's chart, she had *three* tampons inserted at the time of her examination. Her discharge instructions included a recommendation to use sanitary pads or keep a written reminder if she used tampons in the future.

Nice to Meet You for What She Thinks is the First Time

A male patient came to the desk with a blood red face and tears in his eyes.

"What's going on right now?"

He hesitated, which brought me to the conclusion that it had something to do with his genitals or rear end.

"I need to see a doctor," he mumbled.

"What seems to be the problem?"

"I, uh, have something..."

He looked away, embarrassed.

"Trust me," I told the man, "we've seen just about everything there is to see here."

He relaxed, but just slightly. "I have something stuck around my, uh..."

I nodded. "Okay, let's just get you in the system. There's nobody in front of you, so it shouldn't be too long of a wait."

I didn't ask any questions, but I learned a few minutes later that the patient had been 'curious' (at 4 in the morning, and I took that to mean there was probably alcohol involved) to see if a size 2 flat washer would fit around his member. Well, it kind of did, until it became stuck.

Luckily, the cutters stayed in the cabinet. I

guess a nurse just lubed the area up and the washer slipped right off.

The patient didn't make eye contact with me as he left, and the nurses in back said he was so mortified that he really didn't say much to them.

See, that's not the kicker here.

I work overnight shifts, which means there's a whole world of people doing everyday things while I'm sleeping, like, I don't know, grocery shopping, working day shift, performing normal activities that I miss because I'm conked out.

So, as far as I was aware, my day-shift-working friend was still single. I hadn't had a chance to catch up with her for a few days, and I didn't figure much had changed.

Ha ha.

We agreed to meet up at the county fair. She wanted to introduce me to a "super nice, finally *normal*" guy she'd just started dating.

When the former patient and I met face-to-face, he quickly averted his eyes and turned red. My friend knew something was up, but HIPAA kept me from mentioning his ER visit, and I don't think I would ever heart to tell my friend, anyway.

The two didn't work out, and I don't really know what happened to the guy, but I'm hoping he better chose what to experiment with after his trip to our department.

More Inclined to Trust the Kid

A woman arrived carrying a toddler. Her older son was following her.

"What seems to be the problem tonight?" I asked.

It was 2:30 in the morning, so I figured one of the kids woke up with an earache or vomiting.

The woman pointed to her older child. "He's been having a stomachache."

"No I haven't," the boy declared.

"Shh," she told him.

"But my belly doesn't hurt."

"He woke me up and said it hurt."

"*You* woke *me* up," the about-eight-year-old stated, growing irritated.

The patient's mom shook her head and we finished the registration process. I told her to please have a seat in the waiting room. She leaned over the counter and asked, "Do you think they can give me a pregnancy test while they're checking him out?"

Road Trip

A mental health patient was brought in by the cops. They had draped a jacket over her in attempts to cover her near-nudity, as she presented wearing only a pair of granny panties.

The patient was exceptionally quiet. Her appearance was disheveled: her long hair was matted, she had dark circles under her eyes, and it was clear, by the body odor that lingered in the hallway, that she had not bathed in some time.

According to the officers, the patient was picked up from a busy highway, where she was walking in one of the lanes. After doing a bit of backtracking, the cops found the patient's car four miles from where she was found. It was parked on the side of the road and three of her doors were left open.

Not much besides the patient's name and address were known, both gathered from a driver's license officers found in the patient's car. According to the license, the patient lived in Oregon, so Ohio was far from home for her.

Once the patient was seen by staff, her story became more clear. She told nurses and several counselors that she was cooking dinner one evening, when she felt strongly that someone was about to break in her house and kill her, so she grabbed her wallet, got in the car, and just started driving.

At first, the patient said, she didn't know where she would go. But about halfway through her three-day trip, she had decided to try to get to Maine. She would then take a ferry to Canada, where she would live because she 'liked the accents' and 'heard it was easy to hide there.'

Hospital staff called the patient's local police department, hoping to learn more about the patient. Neither party could disclose too much information, but the town from which the patient had come was well aware that she'd disappeared, and it was somewhat big news because when the patient vacated her residence, she forgot to turn off the stove's burners and her house burned down. Neighbors saw the flames, called the fire department, and the patient's husband left work early to see his residence aflame.

Law enforcement confirmed the patient had a long-standing history of mental illness and they had been looking for the patient, but they-or her spouse-never had any idea that she would make it that far from home.

The patient was an ED to mental health until her family could arrange to pick her up.

<u>Once Bitten, Twice Shy...</u>

So, on one of my shifts, I learned I probably wouldn't make a very good babysitter.

A middle-aged woman came to the desk with a once-white dishtowel wrapped around her forearm. Blood had soaked through and she had rotated the towel several times before she finally tied it around a wound I couldn't see at the time of registration.

When I asked the patient what was wrong, she stated she was bitten. Because it was busy and I (apparently stupidly) assumed the bite came from an animal, I simply marked her diagnosis as: 'bite to forearm' and told her to take a seat in the waiting room.

A nurse from the back ER called the patient several minutes later, and because triage was occupied, the woman was taken straight to a room—a non trauma room. Nothing seemed out of place. I figured the patient would require a few stitches, maybe a few rabies shots, and would be out in no time. Again, assuming all of this was my problem.

Almost an hour later, after the patient was transferred to a trauma room, I went to the back to finishing gathering the patient's information. A man I recognized to be a surgeon was exiting her room just as I was walking in, and I immediately was dying to know what was going on. Upon entering the room, I noticed there was a rather large chunk of flesh missing from the patient's arm, leaving her bloodied tendons exposed.

"Wow," I exclaimed. "That must have been one angry animal to have taken that kind of bite out of you."

The patient, calm and collected, appeared confused. "This?" she said sweetly. "Oh, honey, I was babysitting my seven-year-old nephew and when I told him he couldn't have another cookie, he bit me."

It took me a few seconds to catch my breath. I was trying to remember how what grade a seven-year-old would be in. Five, I was thinking, was around kindergarten, so would seven be around first or second grade? And then I remembered being in first and second grade. The rules were about the same: no hitting, no name-calling, and definitely no biting.

"A *kid* did this to you?" I asked in loud surprise.

She nodded, as if her injury was a common one.

"What did you do? I mean, did you spank him?"

"Honey," she exclaimed, appalled by my question, "a good babysitter would know a child of that age couldn't possibly understand the consequences of his actions."

19

For a few minutes after leaving the patient's room, I felt a twinge of shame for my thoughts, but it wore off. I still wonder if the patient feels the same way after her transfer to another hospital for a skin graft.

No Ifs, Ands, or Butts

An ambulance brought in a local college kid. Apparently, the girl and her roommate had been involve in a 'prank war' with one another. The patient said the pranks started off fairly innocent but quickly escalated. There were no rules, and the winner would be crowned when one party surrendered. As soon as I saw what brought the patient in, I made up my mind that the roommate had won.

It took more than two hours to pry the toilet seat from the girl's butt. Most of this time was spent trying different solutions to dissolve the industrial-strength glue. Nurses had to help the patient use the restroom several times during her visit to the ER, and not because she had to urinate. See, her roommate also laced a chocolate cake with laxatives.

Home Protection

A man was brought in via ambulance for blunt force trauma to his head and ribs, in addition to dog bites on his right calf and left forearm. We heard he was involved in a home invasion, so none of us were feeling too sorry for the young man.

His girlfriend arrived just as the EMTs were getting him settled in a trauma room. Her white tank top had splatters of blood on it and her eyes were puffy and red from crying. I started to think that maybe the report over the radio was wrong. Maybe someone broke into *his* house and he was completely innocent.

That was the wrong assumption, too.

The man's girlfriend was so upset because *she* was the one to inflict most of the man's wounds.

She was asleep when he decided to come over. He tried to get inside, but the door was locked, so when she didn't wake to his knocks, he remembered the back door was loose on its hinges, meaning it could be opened—even if it was locked—by lifting up on the handle and pushing it over a little.

The man wasn't meaning to do any harm to his girlfriend. In fact, she told me he often came over after work, just so he could crawl in bed with her. She meant to give him a key, but she simply hadn't had enough time to get to the store to make a copy.

Well, I guess the man jiggled the door a little too much because it finally fell off its hinges and banged against the wall. Thinking there was an intruder in the house, the girl grabbed a softball bat she kept in her room for protection. While her two rescued German Shepherd mixes were attacking the man, the girl took two swings at him: one to the top of the head, followed by another to his ribs. Once she realized she was basically beating the crap out of her boyfriend, she dropped the bat and called the dogs off. Her very next move was calling 911.

In the end, the man ended up with two cracked ribs and a pretty bad concussion. He was kept overnight for observation and ended up with 19 stitches to close up the dog bite wounds.

I thought the sweetest part of the story was that he didn't really seem upset with his girlfriend. He seemed proud that she could take care of herself.

She said she was going to get an extra key made the day the man was discharged.

Old Enough to Know Better...Right?

A patient in her late 40s came to the front desk with her aging mother. Her father, preoccupied with an iPad, stated he would be sitting in the waiting room until the patient's examination was finished.

"What seems to be the problem?" I asked the patient.

She was doubled over in the wheelchair her mother had grabbed for her.

"I'm hurting. I'm hurting so bad."

I nodded. "And where does it hurt?"

She hesitated briefly. "My stomach and down there."

The patient pointed to her pelvic region.

"Well, let's get you in the system," I told her.

"You need to hurry," her mother urged. "She's never been in so much pain."

I glimpsed at my tracking board and then back to the patient. "There seem to be about two patients in front of you. If you'd like to take a spot in the waiting room, it shouldn't be too terribly long until we can get you back."

The patient and her mother thanked me and went to the waiting room to join dad.

I didn't pay much attention to the patient or her family. Traffic picked up within a few minutes of her arrival, and I was running back and forth between the back and front to register patients and finish overnight reports.

After an hour of working on said reports, I looked up to the tracking board and told myself I really *should* go to the back to finish the registration process on two patients. If I printed a face sheet, I could jot down any changes, edit charts up front, and print new face sheets to the back. It was a much faster process than logging on the computer in the back and dragging my cart around, so, obviously, the other process won out.

I went to the back and finished registering a patient with a 'cold and flu symptoms' diagnosis.

As soon as I left that room, I checked the cameras aimed toward the ER front doors. The lobby was empty.

I hurried to the next room.

The patient was curled in a fetal position on her white-paper-lined bed. Her mother worriedly picked at dry skin on her palms.

I formally introduced myself and continued with the registration process.

Nothing really stuck out. The patient was divorced and she told me she was forced to live with her parents after the life-changing event. She worked locally and readily gave her insurance information. She didn't say anything weird or do anything that would stay in my mind...Not then, anyway.

I went back to the front desk.

Two more hours passed, before the triage nurse emerged from the back, cackling uncontrollably. She clamped her hands over her mouth and went to the area behind the registration desk, where she plopped down in an office chair and tried to breathe evenly to rid her beet red complexion.

"Something funny?" I asked as I walked to the back area to gather paperwork.

She tried to nod, but couldn't.

I couldn't laugh. I couldn't frown. I had no idea what was going on.

"That patient, in twelve?"

I nodded. "Yeah? She seemed to be in a lot of pain when she came in. What happened?"

The triage nurse wheezed.

"She asked Wanda if she could see the doctor. And when the doc went in..."

She choked on her chuckles.

The nurse continued, "Get this: this patient said she's been lonely since the divorce."

"So," said the nurse, "she went out and bought a *toy* to help pass the time."

I shrugged. "Okay."

"Well, she said she bought a new toy and decided to use it for the first time tonight."

I nodded for the nurse to continue.

She could hardly speak.

"She said she wanted to try something new

26

and is here because she...She shoved the thing inside of her so deep and hard that her stomach hurts."

The patient, apparently, got carried away with the euphoric sensation she felt with her new toy and shoved a 13-inch toy up inside of herself.

Shortly after her confession, she was diagnosed with pelvic trauma and was ordered to pelvic rest for a week, with a physician's recommendation that she find a smaller toy or not get so excited with the one she had.

Humor in the Hospital

There's nothing funny about a wife walking in our doors and leaving a widow. There's nothing funny about a husband draping himself over his wife's body and sobbing, wondering how he's going to explain to their two-year-old that mommy isn't coming home. When a baby comes in unresponsive and with blue lips because she somehow found and drank drain cleaner, nobody's laughing.

These were real cases.

Three people, at various points on the line of life, died. Hearts broke. Family members fainted. Thoughts went from cook outs to funeral arrangements in a matter of seconds following that news none of us ever want anyone to hear.

Some things we see, though, *are* funny, and that's okay. I don't just tell this to myself to feel like a better person for giggling about some of the things I've seen. Laughter in this job, in this field, is necessary for survival. If you can't take a minute to at least smile, the bad things you see, hear, feel...those feelings of hopelessness and grief and questioning faith will eat you alive and spit you out without hesitation.

The fact is, when patients walk through these doors, they are each treated in the highest regard, no matter their race, mental status, 'net worth', age, or physical appearance. Treatment isn't different based on street smarts versus book smarts. Whether or not a patient has insurance, is on public assistance, or pays more money to a well-known insurance company than most of us make in a year doesn't matter; a patient will receive the best care possible. A nurse won't look at you and say, "Well, it's clear that you haven't showered in a week and your shoes are falling apart, so since you can't afford the bill, we're not treating you."

And I have to say, stupidity, nastiness, rudeness...It doesn't matter if people are rich, poor, black, blue, purple...We're *all* capable of doing stupid things, myself included.

There's no prejudice when it comes to this job. There **can't** be. There's no shortage of respect offered to patients at this hospital. I don't know what happens at other hospitals, but I can almost guarantee *every* health professional you speak with will have at least one memorable funny story about his or her career. It doesn't mean we don't care or that we think poorly of our patients.

The ER Express-Patching You Up in 30 Minutes or Less

A woman ran inside, wearing a velour jogging suit. Her hair and makeup were flawless. It was close to four in the morning and she had more pep in her than any of my coworkers at that time. I mean, you don't know what miserable is until four or five in the morning hits on an overnight shift and you start to question your entire life. (*'What did I do to get here?' Why did I volunteer to take Michelle's shift?' 'The word 'the'...is that spelled right? T-h-e. I think that's right, but maybe I should look it up.' 'I get to go home in two hours. I'll close my eyes for 10 minutes and...look at that, only eight seconds have passed.'*)

"I called you," she said, bugging her eyes, as if that was all I needed to know.

This wasn't the first time I've heard this.

"You must have spoken to a unit clerk or a nurse in the back. What seems to be the problem this morning?"

She paced and breathed hard. "I've been having chest pain for about an hour." She frowned and gave an irritated laugh. "And you know what? I don't have time for this crap, I really don't."

The security guard sitting next to me moved at

record speed to get the woman a wheelchair. He was primarily a day-shift guard and was working his first overnight shift in over a year. Throughout the night, it was clear he seemed to have forgotten that a different group of crazy comes out when the sun goes down.

"I'm not sitting," she argued. "I'm telling you, I *really* don't have time for this."

"Ma'am," I said, as I dialed the charge nurse's number, "they're going to put you in a chair when they come for you. It's just hospital policy for heart complaints."

She huffed and puffed. I told the charge nurse we had a chest pain up front, to which she replied someone was on the way.

"How long will this take? I have stuff to do today. I have to make sure the kids are up for school, have a tanning appointment at eight..."

"It could take a while," the guard answered because I was too dumbfounded to reply.

"The nurse on the phone promised I could be out of here in 30 minutes or less."

The patient signed out AMA after her EKG came back with abnormal results. She said she just couldn't waste her time at the hospital because she had too many appointments that day, including getting her Pomeranian to the groomer "for a bath and new bows."

I went in early the next evening and saw the patient's name on the tracking board. She was being admitted to Critical Care after she went to

Cath Lab for a stent. I guess she had time to come in after making all of her appointments.

Pay it Forward

It was another busy overnight shift on day three of my nine-day stretch of shifts before I was supposed to get one day off, and I was drowning in a mess of paperwork I didn't have the time to organize.

There were three consecutive patients I had registered to send to OB for labor checks, and I was trying to keep track of all the bed transfers and direct admits to floors so I could get it all out of the way, once the patients in the lobby were admitted to the ER.

A young male—the last patient in a long line—approached the registration desk. He seemed jittery.

"I need to talk to someone," he told me.

There were scabs on his cheeks and forehead. Judging by his disheveled appearance and wound-up behavior, I figured he wanted to see a mental health counselor.

Nope.

"So my girlfriend was diagnosed with a yeast infection, like, two days ago," he started. "It was bad. Really bad. Like, it was just not good at all."

He seemed distant by the tone of his voice, as if he wasn't serious. I bit my lip and wondered what he would say next. He looked to me for a

33

reply.

"Okay."

"Well," he continued, "last night, she and I participated in oral sex with each other."

The security guard standing next to me shot me a look, asking me if the patient was being truthful. I still felt like he just came in to mess with me, maybe as a prank. After all, move-in-day at the local college was two nights before, and he was the perfect age to be involved in some silly dare proposed by goofy peers.

"Okay," I said.

He hovered his open palm over his face.

"Well now I have all these splotches on my face and my throat hurts, and I'm pretty sure I caught her yeast infection."

"Ooo-kay."

He motioned to his face again. "So, yeah. I'm here because I have a yeast infection on my face. And it all happened because I was giving my girlfriend oral sex."

I signed the patient in and directed him to the packed waiting room.

It turns out that the patient *did* test positive for yeast growth on his face, and he was diagnosed with thrush. He was told to abstain from oral sex until his girlfriend's yeast infection cleared up.

The one word going around after that? "Ewwwwwww."

The Choices We Make

Sadly, in this area (and so many others), methamphetamine production is a concern and a problem that plagues not only drug abusers, but farmers, families, and law enforcement officers.

Four ambulances pulled in the bay a little after two in the morning and there was already heavy chatter and a sense of urgency before the vehicles even arrived with the patients. Nurses were dressed in protective gear and the decontamination room was ready to go, complete with towels and gowns stacked to the side.

At the time, I didn't have an idea of what was going on or bother to ask.

EMTs rolled in patients one by one. I watched on the cameras as three of the patients flopped around on their stretchers like fish out of water. They were shrieking and sobbing. The patient on the last stretcher didn't move. I leaned in closer to the camera when I noticed the paramedics were in no hurry to move the patient. It became clear to me that the patient was dead.

A nurse came to the front and took a seat in the back part of the office. She placed her palms against her face and cried.

"What's wrong?" I asked.

She shook her head. "This one is just, uh,

hitting me pretty hard."

"What's going on?"

She sniffled and pulled her hands away from her face. Her cheeks were red and her makeup was smudged.

"They're just so young."

She returned to sobbing and I left her alone to work through her feelings.

Three names popped up on the tracking board, each with a diagnosis of 'chemical exposure' and burns to various body parts.

It didn't immediately come to me, what happened to bring these teenagers to the ER with the diagnoses at hand. If I was thinking anything, it still had nothing to do with drugs.

EMTs came to the desk, asking for face sheets on the patients. That's when they told me the story.

Paramedics were called to a gravel road just outside of town, where they found a banged-up car. It had rolled twice and came to rest in a ditch.

The driver hadn't hit a deer or gone off the road when changing a radio station.

Four teenagers were speeding away from a farm, where they had stolen two tanks filled with anhydrous ammonia. One of the teens, a male, sat in the passenger seat and held one of the containers on his lap. In the backseat, it was a similar set up.

And everything was fine, I guess, until the tank the front seat passenger was holding exploded. His skin shriveled up. Luckily, he had managed to close his eyes, but a drop of the chemicals splashed his eyeball and the tighter he closed his eyes, the more it burned.

When the tank exploded, the driver crashed the car. According to the paramedics, one of the survivors said the second tank of ammonia exploded when the car rolled for the first time. By the second roll, everyone in the vehicle had been subjected to chemical burns and injuries sustained from the wreck.

Paramedics said the driver died en route to the ER.

The other three patients were life-lined to a hospital specializing in burns. The front-seat passenger sustained burns primarily to his face and chest. He still comes to the ER for diagnoses related to the accident and said he was told he'll never look 'normal' again. He's blind in one eye, but thankful for his life and wants to travel to high schools to speak about the event. Unfortunately, his health isn't in the best condition for him to do so, but he hopes one day soon it will be.

One of the other two survivors died a few days after the accident.

Creepy Crawlies

I don't know what it is, exactly, about human psychology, but I've noticed most of my coworkers feel itchy after dealing with patients presenting with scabies or fleas or even poison ivy. I'm not exempt from this. I go overboard on sanitizing the counter, pens, clipboard—anything the patient *may* have touched. I wash my hands repeatedly, check my clothes, and still end up doing the 'ER full body squirm' a few times throughout the night.

One night, we were *all* doing that squirm.

After having a crazy night that never seemed like it was going to end, everything came to a halt and it was so quiet in the lobby that you could hear a pin drop. I—and all of my coworkers—took the opportunity to race to the bathrooms around the hospital, unsure of when the next opportunity would present itself.

I knew that moment of silence was too good to be true. Just as soon as I started to unzip my pants, I heard a patient screaming.

"Hello? Is anyone going to help me or not?"

"Just a second," I called.

I groaned and mumbled a few choice words under my breath, but I left that bathroom with the sweetest smile on my face.

"How can we help you tonight?"

"I was out here for ten minutes," the patient yelled. "I came all the way over here from 123 Alphabet Drive, and then I have to wait? I'm having an emergency."

I wanted to roll my eyes, but it was clear the patient was agitated.

"What's the problem tonight?" I asked, hoping I could register the patient and return to the restroom.

He held out both arms and rotated them. The man had large, bleeding welts spotting his skin.

"Okay," I replied, "let's register you."

"Just take me back to a room," he screamed at me.

I gave a hard stare to the security office's two-way mirror, hoping one of the guards would take notice and come out to the lobby. The patient grew increasingly angry with every question I asked him, to the point I thought he was going to hit me when he raised the clipboard. Instead, he slammed it on the counter.

"I'm calling the nurse now," I told the man. "I just have to get your labels from the printer, okay?"

He instantly changed his attitude but it didn't last long. From the time it took me to get to the printer and copy his signature sheet, which maybe took a whole eight seconds, the man was screaming again. I left his paperwork atop the copier and went to the open office space behind the registration desk.

I dialed security and asked one of the guards to please sit near me while the patient was in the lobby.

When the guard emerged, the patient appeared calm. He and the guard talked a bit about the weather before the triage nurse called his name.

He didn't last 10 seconds in the triage seat before he was screaming at the triage nurse. The patient couldn't understand why his vital signs were important to the reason of his visit, and the nurse had to repeat her questions three or four times each just to get the patient to shout an answer.

Finally, the security guard stepped in and told the patient to settle down. He apologized, but then started screaming at the guard.

"I am covered in bugs," the patient screeched.

I hadn't seen any bugs on the patient when he arrived. The triage nurse apparently couldn't see them, either.

"They're right here," he argued.

"Sir," the nurse stated, "you're picking at scabs right now."

I figured the patient was on drugs.

The nurse took the patient back to a room, just so she could have a few seconds to regroup. She soon hurried to the front and pointed at the phone.

"Call housekeeping and start wiping down your stuff."

"Why?" I questioned.

"When he sat down on the bed back there,"

the nurse explained, "bugs just started dropping off of him, like *pouring* off of him like you'd see in the movies. He has bed bugs, and he has them bad."

Housekeeping arrived and sprayed the lobby. I scrubbed the counter and everything the patient had remotely come close to. The triage nurse asked me to help her inspect her area.

She and I were already itching. She went to the locker room and I went to the bathroom, where we disrobed and shook out our clothes.

When I came out of the bathroom, the patient was walking out the door. He would have left without incident, I think, but he saw me and then started ranting and raving again.

"This hospital is horrible. All I wanted was someone to come to my house and get rid of the bugs. That's why you're here."

I still suspected the patient was on drugs.

He came back three more times that night. The room he was originally in was put on isolation by housekeeping each time he eloped. He was eventually told he'd have to stay for treatment or leave.

So far, we haven't seen the patient again, but we start feeling itchy whenever someone brings him up.

Die the Way You Live

An older woman helped a man into a wheelchair and pushed him to the registration desk.

"What's going on right now?" I asked.

"My genius husband fell off the roof and now we think he's broken a few bones."

He shook his head. "Nope. I probably just cracked a few ribs, maybe sprained my ankle."

"When did you fall off the roof?" I asked with raised brows. I quickly glanced at the clock.

He shrugged. "About twenty minutes ago."

"What were you doing on the roof at three in the morning?" I exclaimed.

He started to speak, but his wife cut him off. "I told you, he's a genius. He decided cleaning the gutters couldn't wait, since that big storm is supposed to come in soon."

I slowly nodded, with my eyes widened and my mouth hanging open. "Right."

"He's always doing stuff like this. It's going to be the way he goes out, too. I can just feel it."

"Woman," the patient nagged, "I already told you, I'm going to leave this world doing what I love best: fishing and drinking beer."

I chuckled, registered the patient, and later watched him leave. He was partly right. He suffered from cracked ribs, but he did break his ankle.

Some time later, I was sitting at switchboard, relieving the operator so she could take her break. I thumbed through a newspaper she had on the desk.

There was the former patient, his name in bold above a gray scale picture of his smiling face.

According to the article, the patient took a fall from his roof while he was nailing down a few loose shingles. This time, he wasn't so lucky to make it to the ER. His obituary called for a celebration of life, rather than dwelling on sadness, and I still think of the patient every now and then. Wherever he is, I hope he's doing what he loved best: fishing and drinking beer.

Bible Thumper

After sending a newly-registered patient to the waiting room, I looked up at the camera at just the right time and saw she was smacking her arm with a book.

Concerned, I called the charge nurse.

When confronted about her behavior, the patient responded, "My mom told me this cyst will go away if I hit it with a bible."

You know it's going to be a fun night when you're walking into work and pass six cop cars, two discharged patients arguing over how they're going to divvy up the pills they were just prescribed, and a patient wandering around the parking lot with his (very open) gown on backwards.

When Big Brother is After You

A young patient presented to the ER with lacerations to her forehead, cheeks, neck, forearms, hands, and abdomen. Most of the cuts appeared to be shallow, but all were bleeding or had bled enough to leave streaks of blood on the patient's skin and clothes. There were multiple bruises on her face and arms. She was sobbing and clinging to an older woman she identified as one of her sisters.

The patient couldn't speak much. A nurse came out and took her to the back in hopes of relaxing her rapid breathing, leaving the sister to register the patient.

"What exactly happened?" I asked. "Was she in a fight?"

"Her husband did this," the woman stated bitterly. "Because she told him she's pregnant."

She continued to explain that the patient's husband repeatedly kicked the patient in the stomach and then told her he was going to kill her because it was the only way to make sure he 'wouldn't have another kid to owe child support to.' The patient managed to crawl away long enough to call her sister for help, but the patient's husband kicked down the bathroom door. He was dragging her through the living room by her hair when her sister arrived. The patient's sister attempted to pull the man from the patient, but he punched her in the face multiple times before leaving the home.

I didn't have anything to say back, really, besides, "They'll help you file a police report in the back."

The sister nodded. "Oh, they're already on the way. I made sure to call them on the way here. You might be seeing her husband tonight, too, because our brother went out looking for him. He'd better hope the cops get him first."

The patient experienced a miscarriage and was placed upstairs for observation. Her sister stayed with her and an officer offered to check in with the two throughout the night.

We did see the patient's husband a few hours later. EMTs rolled him inside on a stretcher and a trauma code was activated due to his 11 broken bones, a head injury, and a collapsed lung. He refused to name his assailant.

Sadly, domestic violence against both men and women is common in the ER, but resources are available. If you or anyone you know need help, call the National Domestic Violence Hotline at 1-800-799-SAFE (7233), or visit their website: http://www.thehotline.org/ .

Oh, So That's What That's For

A patient was brought in via ambulance with a chief complaint of 'menstrual cramps.' Because the patient's daughter was three-years-old and couldn't be left alone, EMTs let the child ride up front with them and told the patient they could wait at the hospital with the child for 30 minutes, until the patient could call her mother to come for the child.

Well, 30 minutes passed, and the EMTs discovered the patient never called her mother. She never intended to call her, and she refused to contact anyone else for childcare. She said she 'didn't want to bother anyone.'

Yeah, well, the patient kicked and screamed and shouted when EMTs told her they had to go and wanted to child to return to the patient's room—where the patient was eating a meal she had requested and was watching television.

The patient screamed out, "Just leave her with a nurse. My Medicaid will pay them for watching her."

Patient's Daughter: I want to know why that person was taken back before my mom. We've been waiting out here for twenty minutes, and then someone comes in, and you guys took him back first. That's not fair. We were first, and I demand we be seen in the order we check in.

My Coworker: Ma'am, we took that patient back because it's a trauma case.

Patient's Daughter: Well, my mom is in a lot of pain and needs to be seen *now*. How do you know you won't have to amputate her leg?

The patient presented with an ingrown hair and once she was seen, she was discharged 10 minutes later. The other patient was transferred to another hospital after he presented with his ulna being completely snapped in half.

You Mean I Have to Stay?

A woman brought in a small child to be seen for vomiting and cold/flu symptoms. She seemed to be irritated that the babysitter called her and interrupted a night out.

Triage called the patient's name and mom encouraged the child to go with the nurse.

"How long do you think this is going to take?" asked his mother.

The nurse shrugged. "It can sometimes take a few hours, depending on what lab finds and how he'll react to medicine. We'll have to monitor his fever for a while, too."

Mom smiled. "Okay. Well, I gave my number to the girl at the front desk, so if you could call me when you're finished, someone will be here to pick him up."

She started to walk away.

I know my facial expression showed a look of shock. At first, I couldn't tell if the woman was serious, but figured she was when she was almost to the door.

"Ma'am," firmly stated the triage nurse, "you can't leave him here without parental supervision."

Mom was mad. The patient was in the ER for two hours, during which time I estimated mom was outside, smoking and talking on her cell phone for about an hour and a half of it.

A patient came to the ER with his highly-concerned girlfriend. He said he was suffering from an acne outbreak on his genitals.

"I even gave some some Stridex pads to use," the girlfriend said, "but they didn't help much."

They didn't help much because the patient didn't have acne. He had herpes he contracted from his *other* girlfriend.

Me: Can you sign the consent form for me tonight?

Frequent Patient: No. I can't see.

ER Tech: Open your eyes, then!

The patient opened her eyes, signed my paper, and then went on to try the act for the next person to enter her room.

Held Hostage

One evening, a family came in with a baby to be seen. Because only two visitors are allowed in back (with exception to a dying patient or someone waiting to be admitted to a floor), three of the family's friends sat in the waiting room.

Now, our doors are set up in an odd way. Only one of the three-panel-glass doors open. We often see patients and/or visitors approach the wrong end of the door, realize the mistake, and leave through the proper side.

A younger woman stood at the stationary end of the door.

I watched her for a few seconds and assumed she would try the other end.

Yeah, no.

"You have to go to the other side," I called out to her.

She pouted.

"This is illegal, you know," she spat at me.

She returned to the waiting room. We were busy, so I didn't think much of the moment. The woman shrugged and took a seat in the waiting room with her friend. They whispered to one another for a long time and occasionally got up from their seats to look down the hall. At one point, the girl tried to get through the locked double doors at the end of the hall, but after a certain time, that part of the hospital is off limits without a pass. She never asked for a pass, and I never asked if she wanted one.

An **hour** later, the woman's friend approached the registration desk.

"Excuse me?" he asked me. "Can you tell me where the closest exit is?"

I was confused. He entered the ER with his friend, and it was kind of difficult to miss the big red 'EXIT' sign over the doors.

I pointed to the front doors. "Uh, there."

"But isn't that locked? My friend said we can't go out those doors because they're locked, that we have to go to the other side of the hospital. But the other doors are locked, too."

Seriously?

"Uh," I hesitated. "She was standing in front of the part of the door that doesn't move."

He rolled his eyes. "She's so dumb."

The gentleman returned to the waiting room. Judging by the response of the young woman, she was embarrassed half to death.

The two walked to the (right) side of the door and exited the hospital to make phone calls. They returned a few minutes later and went back to the waiting room.

The rest of the patient's family emerged from the back part of the ER.

Instead of asking how the patient was doing,

the guy blurted out, "You know your daughter doesn't know how to work an automatic door, right?"

"I'm sorry I'm so stupid," she laughed.

According to the patient's family member, she believed we were trying to keep her inside.

Not A Christmas Story

It was July 4th and we expected the day shift to be busy. Most of us figured that the evening shift would be slower than usual, just because most people in the area would be watching fireworks. Then, we figured, the overnight shift would be the ER experiencing the real rush of the holiday: firework injuries, heat exhaustion, and intoxication.

Some of us were starting to wonder if we would see a firework injury. It was pushing 11 and we'd only seen a few for the entire month of July so far, all of which were superficial scratches or burns no worse than accidentally touching a curling iron for a whole millisecond.

And around that time is when our outdoor 'Emergency Button' was pushed. The Emergency Button is a big red button on the outer wall of the ER. Its primary function is to alert staff of any losses of limbs, severe bleeding, chemical exposure, and/or inability to make it inside without assistance. Several people have hit it before—both on purpose and also accidentally—but nobody's ever *really* needed help; they just 'wanted to see' what would happen.

The unit clerk called and asked in a tired tone,

"Did a kid just hit the button?"

I stood and peered outside the best I could. A woman was holding a bloody towel over a teenage girl's face and a man was trying to hold the girl upright.

"Nope," I said to the unit clerk. "You should send someone out here. Hurry."

Two nurses rushed out from the back and helped the teen and her parents inside. The entire family panicked and couldn't express what had happened.

"Let me see," one of the nurses said to the girl. She pried mom's grip from the towel to check out the injury.

The teen's right eyeball was hanging out of its socket.

Other patients in the lobby—either leaving or registering—gasped, the over-exaggerated gasps you hear in movies.

Nurses rushed the girl and her family back to a trauma room.

According to the family, the teenager's eye was pierced by a runaway bottle rocket. They tried to pull the firework from her ruptured globe, but it was stuck. Before they knew it, one of the parents yanked hard on the firework and pulled her eyeball out with it.

Even before being heavily medicated, the patient was rather calm, mostly from shock, I think. She was transferred to another hospital with the understanding that she would lose her eye at a young age of 17.

"You could literally put a box of rocks on the counter and label it 'food,' and we would try to eat them because telling our fall risk patient for the nine-hundredth time to stop trying to get out of bed wipes us out and leaves us starving." --*An RN, on ER staff eating habits.*

The People You Meet

The shift in question started off slowly but, as it usually happens, all hell broke loose out of nowhere. Three ambulances pulled in the bay and the lobby became flooded with impatient visitors and people waiting to be seen by a doctor. I separated the crowd by those waiting to be seen versus those waiting for a pass to visit patients in the rest of the hospital and visitors for rooms in the back.

After registering four patients for the ER, I started calling people forward to see if they could go back to visit.

The first three visitors didn't have much of a story to go along with them. I was hoping none of them would have a story, honestly, because I was the only registration clerk there and I wanted everything to play out smoothly until 7:05 came along and I could clock out.

Yeah, nope.

Just as a male approached the desk, I could hear a patient shrieking and squalling.

"You're here to visit?" I asked the man, trying hard to ignore the continuous cries from the patient in the back.

He nodded. "I'm here to see the girl screaming."

"Are you related?"

He nodded again and sighed. "She's my daughter. They just brought her on the ambulance. She decided to have a one-person party while my wife and I were gone, so we came home to her passed out on the kitchen floor."

"Oh, wow," I stated, expressing genuine concern. The man didn't appear to be *that* old. I wondered how old his daughter was, but I didn't ask and didn't have to. Her name and age quickly appeared on my tracking board. She wasn't even in her teen years yet.

Dad signed the consent form and agreed to answer registration questions while the EMTs and nurses were situating the patient in her room.

I glanced up to the security camera monitors and saw the EMTs wheeling out an empty stretcher. Just as I picked up the phone to call the ER unit clerk, the man's daughter let out a string of obscenities that would put a foul-mouthed sailor to shame. A flustered nurse ran through the double doors to the left of the counter and was clearly out of breath.

"Do we have family for room five yet?" she asked me. "We really need some help trying to get this patient to calm down."

The patient's father shook his head. "I guess I'll claim her."

"You're dad?" asked the nurse.

The man nodded. "I don't know for how much longer, though, because I might have to disown the little hellion," he joked.

I thought dad being in the room would encourage the patient to behave better, but I've been wrong a lot lately.

Instead of the patient's father's presence calming her, it only seemed to feed her anger. She continued screeching at the top of her lungs and I'm pretty sure she shouted every bad word in existence.

Patients kept flooding in. Nobody could ignore the screams and everyone seemed to have a theory on what was going on in the back.

"Someone must be hurt pretty bad."

"Boy, she doesn't sound happy."

"I bet she has a kidney stone. That's what I sounded like when I had one."

Security was paged to the patient's room in a desperate attempt to persuade the girl to relax. I ran to the back to drop off paperwork and saw a seven-months-pregnant nurse cringing and scrubbing the front of her scrub top with a wet rag.

"Did she spit on you?" the doctor asked her.

The nurse's nostrils flared and she gritted her teeth. "She flung her vomit bag at me."

The doctor nodded and thought for a minute before he shrugged and said, "Okay, get the cuffs."

'The cuffs' aren't generally brought out in this ER. Most patients displaying aggression are brought in by police officers and are restrained using real handcuffs. Other out of control patients often calm down after security arrives or nurses threaten to call the police. Every now and then, though, black canvas restraints are brought out of storage and are used to keep a patient's arms and legs cuffed to the bed rails.

I stayed out of the mess and went back up front, but it was obvious that staff members were attempting to apply the restraints when the patient's shrieks grew in volume and her cursing sped up.

A few minutes later, two city police officers arrived. I knew the nurses were desperate to calm the patient without the use of sedatives. Security generally refuses to touch a patient unless there is an emergency situation when it becomes unavoidable.

The patient continued shouting.

"You need to calm down," I heard an officer order loudly.

The triage nurse walked to my side and whispered to me, "Did her dad tell you how much she drank?"

I shook my head as I thumbed through my messy pile of face sheets.

"She drank a jar of moonshine and half a bottle of Merlot. That kid is plastered right now."

I was shocked at what the nurse told me, but mostly because I couldn't understand how a pre-teen could consume so much alcohol and still be conscious enough to be screaming her head off.

Another squad car pulled up and parked outside the Emergency Room entrance and I wondered to myself how many adults it would take to get the patient to knock it off.

Two officers escorted a cuffed man to the registration desk. He towered over me and gasped for air as if he had just participated in a marathon.

"Is this a drug screen or a medical clearance?" I asked a female officer.

"Neither," she replied. "He's going to the psych floor because he wants to harm himself."

"Okay," I nodded.

"He's dripping blood," the officer informed me. "He cut his wrist up, but I had to cuff it because he's violent."

I glanced to the patient.

He gave a sweet, closed-lipped smile. "I won't hurt you."

I ignored the patient's remark and registered him.

"It's going to be a minute," I told the officer. "I can't send you back to a room because I don't know which one the triage nurse needs."

"We're going to see him through triage," the nurse piped up. "They have to get fifteen cleaned while he's up here."

I shrugged to the officers. "I guess you guys can sit on the bench. As soon as she's finished with the patient she's with now, the triage nurse will see you."

It didn't take too long before triage called the newest patient back. While a male officer was escorting the patient to the triage area to be weighed and have his vitals checked, the female officer pulled me to the side.

"Do you know what this guy did to be here?"

"Besides cut himself up?" I asked with raised brows.

"He stabbed his dog," she told me in a heavy whisper.

"What?" I questioned loudly. I lowered my voice. "He, like...really stabbed his dog?"

She nodded. "He said he was watching TV and had an urge to kill something, so I guess he just leaned over and stabbed the dog."

"Oh my."

The officer continued, "There was blood all over this guy's apartment. The dog was trying to get away. And I guess, you know, after the guy did it, he used the same knife to start slicing at himself."

I felt sick to my stomach. "Did you guys leave the dog there to die?"

"No," she explained. "We have animal control going in to take it to an emergency vet."

"Was it bad?"

"I'm surprised the dog wasn't dead by the time we got there," she scowled. "But this is what we're dealing with tonight. Nobody is going in his room without us. If you have any other papers for him to sign, bring them to me and I'll sign them. He's not to have a pen."

"Hey," the triage nurse told the male officer, "I need to get these cuffs off to take his vitals. Can we at least get one off?"

The female officer excused herself and pulled her keys from her belt while her partner drew his gun and aimed it at the dog-stabber. The patient complied and never made a move against anyone.

I think it should go without saying that stabbing a dog is pretty much a sure way to get sent to the psychiatric floor, but I still heard nurses asking about the patient the next night. It's been 10 days and the patient is still there. Nobody knows where he's going next.

It's a lot more common than I thought it would be that a 'boyfriend' or 'girlfriend' will bring his/her significant other to the ER, yet can't tell us the patient's last name, birthday, or, sometimes, even first name.

Signs We Really Want to Post

-Standing in the doorway, hallway, or at the desk and staring at me for 20 minutes doesn't make the process going any faster.

-If you're presenting with a 98.9 fever, make yourself comfortable in the waiting room.

-Uh, just because you came in with a friend doesn't mean you have clearance to walk anywhere you please when the urge strikes.

-EMTs: You will get your face sheet as soon as the patient is in the system. Give me more than 30 seconds. BTW, it would be helpful if you could give me a name.

-We ALL work in the same hospital. A patient is coding on ICU, a level 1 I-baby was just born, and the violent patient you just discharged to mental health is clawing her eyes out and needs to be sedated—but can't be, because I have to flip her account first. Let's respect one another. Let's take ONE second to think that we're all doing something to save someone's life.

-Right now, this department has three patients

*over the age of 85 and they're all scared and
alone. Call your parents. Volunteer at a nursing
home.*

*-Please excuse me if I don't type in your
diagnosis of 'headache' in under .002 seconds.
I've been fighting a migraine for two hours and
have nine more to work before I can go home and
try to sleep it off.*

*-If you are remotely interested in inventing,
please start working on an inhaler that dispenses
triple-caffeinated coffee bursts. --Sincerely, the
baby was up, someone knocked on my door, and I
only managed to get 20 minutes of sleep before
this 16-hour shift. P.S. I will test it for free.*

*-Don't tell me your kid's name is 'Megan,' yet
get mad at me because I didn't have a clue that it
would be spelled 'Maeyguin.' Also see: Sorry I
mispronounced the name you obviously made up.
I had no idea I was supposed to pronounce
'Xuhveeair' as Javier, so excuse me for butchering
it. You don't have to yell at me.*

*- "You don't look that bus—." I swear to all
things holy, if you jinx me, I'm going to drag you
by the scruff of your neck to help me do my job.*

*-If you feel your wait time is too long, please
explain to the other eight people in front of you*

that the 'weird brown spot' on your toe needs to be seen before hives, active bleeding, or flank pain.

-The fact that we are employed by this hospital does not mean we are not sometimes bothered by what you present. Please excuse me if I need to pass off your vomiting to someone more comfortable with your bodily functions. Come back when you cut off an arm and blood is spurting all over the place, and I'll be happy to help you.

-He who carries a full urinal down the hall has right-of-way.

-We are all very well aware that you work here, even without you having to tell us 50 times. Even so, expect to wait if you're presenting with something non-critical.

-Wearing scrubs when you accompany your family member to the ER doesn't give you free reign to interrupt the nurse in charge of your family member's care. Remember, if it wasn't an emergency, you could be handling it on your own.

Assume They're All Serious

At three in the morning, a mom brought her seven-year-old son in to be seen.

"He went to a cookout at his dad's house last night and came home with five mosquito bites," the mom angrily stated. "I told my ex to spray him down, but I guess he'll never do what I tell him to do."

I bit my lip and gave a soft nod, nervously trapped before the bitter mom.

"And what seems to be the problem tonight?" I asked.

"Uh," she spat, "he has *five* mosquito bites."

Before leaving home for my shift, I counted 25 on my foot, so I wasn't exactly getting the point. Mosquitoes were bad that year.

"Okay...Are you here for those?"

"Well, *yeah*. I need him to be checked out, to make sure he doesn't have malaria now."

I opened my mouth and blinked at the woman.

"Really?" I asked.

This set the mom off. Yeah, she *was* serious. That woman cussed me up and down and sideways and backways. She was still cussing when the doc discharged her kid 15 minutes later with a suggestion for her to buy the boy some anti-itch cream.

<u>Night of the 912s</u>

The overnight shift was already pretty busy. Summer had officially begun, and the ER was flooded with all kinds of diagnoses, from kids presenting injuries after getting whacked in the nose with baseballs, to adults presenting burns after recklessly playing with fireworks, to parents bringing in mosquito-bitten babies because they were *positive* their newly-out-of-the-womb children had mumps.

I was scrambling to keep up and knew at the beginning of my shift that I wouldn't be able to finish my reports, if I could even start them. I cleared off the front desk and rolled up my sleeves. Thick beads of sweat formed around my hairline and rolled down my forehead as I jogged from the front to the back to gather emergency information on the second stemi patient I'd dealt with in 30 minutes.

When I came back up front, I saw two families coming through the doors, and when I looked to the surveillance monitors to the left, four ambulances had pulled in the bay.

"Why does everyone in this county and all the others wait until I'm working to decide they need medical treatment?" the triage nurse jokingly cried.

I shrugged. "I can't wait to see our numbers

for tonight. They're going to be crazy."

"Well, since you and I've clocked in, we've already seen twenty-two patients. They're calling in some reinforcements."

For this ER, 22 patients in an hour is something amazing, like 'there's been a catastrophic event' amazing. There are plenty of overnights when we don't even handle 22 patients in a single shift. The tracking board was full, the last few vacant beds in back were snatched up by the patients brought in via ambulance, techs were being ordered to stat clean rooms as soon as patients were discharged, and doctors were trying to discharge superficial cases as soon as possible.

Another nurse ran from the back and grabbed a wheelchair. Her hair was a wild, frizzy mess and she was panting.

"Is it a full moon tonight?" she yelled. "What the heck is going on right now?"

She didn't wait around for an answer. She couldn't. That nurse was responsible for two other patients in addition to the one who'd just been marked as discharged, and her remaining patients were rumored to be in critical condition following an MVA, making them immediate 912 traumas.

The way the first hour of the shift was going, it was no surprise that three of the four patients from the ambulances were also 912 traumas. Two were involved in MVAs with each other, while one was listed as an assault. The last patient from the ambulances came in for finger pain.

About 20 minutes had passed. Families arrived for three of those patients, meaning I didn't have to rush to the back and be stuck in a line with x-ray, CT, and lab. A nurse came out from the back and asked if family had arrived for the assault patient. I just shook my head.

"I can come back and get contact information," I offered.

The nurse scoffed. "You're not getting anything from him. He's been beat to a pulp and is highly intoxicated on top of all of that. Only got his name because the cop that arrived on scene just arrested him the other night. We're contacting a flight team now. We really need his family here, since he's a minor. Call me if anyone shows up, huh? And if they do, the *only* person coming back here is mom or dad. Absolutely no exceptions to that until I can talk to a parent, okay?"

The cops came and went. Another half hour had passed before anyone arrived for the patient. At first, it was manageable.

The minor patient's adult cousin confirmed all of his information, but since she was not an immediate family member, she could not sign our consent forms. A doctor spoke to the woman and informed her the patient would soon be transported via helicopter to a hospital a few hours away.

"I'm going to leave and go find his mom," the woman told me.

I nodded and watched her leave.

Two codes were called on the overhead pager.

One was for security to respond to a fight on the OB floor, and another was a Code 99 for a patient on ICU.

I was trying to clear up my working area when the ETOH/assault victim's mother arrived. She could hardly walk straight and was accompanied by a very-pregnant teenage girl.

The girl approached the counter. "I need to see my boyfriend."

"I'm sorry," I said, "but the only visitors the nurse has authorized are parents for right now."

"But I'm his baby mamma. Got one and a half kids with him."

Yes, she actually said that.

She swept blonde hair from her eyes and started making a fist.

"You are going to let me see him. Oh, I don't want to go to jail tonight. Lord help me, I don't want to go to jail."

I sighed and ignored the girl.

"Mom?" I asked of the out-of-it woman behind the teenager.

She nodded and wiped tears from her eyes.

"They really want to see you in the back. Do you think you can sign some forms for me? We already confirmed address and stuff with the first woman a little earlier."

The teenage girl walked off, cursing. She blended in with a crowd of loud teenage boys who came bursting through the front doors.

"I'm gonna kill the person that did this," one

shouted loudly.

I thought about calling security, but knew they were both off dealing with that fight on OB.

The aggressive teenage boy came to the desk and slammed his fist on the counter.

"And what's this about, you not letting her see her old man?"

Mom was of absolutely no help. She'd been signing her name on the consent form the whole time and said nothing to the kids.

"I need you all to go sit down now," I stated firmly.

"No," said the pregnant girlfriend. "What you need to do is let me go see my boyfriend."

The boy who'd slammed his fist on the counter started punching his open left palm. "I'm gonna kill someone tonight. You should let me back there or it's gonna be you."

I picked up the phone and dialed the operator.

"I need you to page security to me as soon as possible," I said.

The group of teenagers erupted into laughter and cynical remarks.

"Gonna call the fake po-po on me?" the boy asked.

Finally, mom spoke up.

"Half of you guys are on probation," she snapped. "Go sit down. It's not this girl's fault you can't get in. We'll take care of it in a few minutes."

Some of the kids went to the waiting room, but the trouble makers, of course, didn't.

Security called just as the patient's nurse popped up at the front.

"I'm going to start by taking mom back," she explained to everyone in the lobby. "Maybe after a while, visitors can come back two at a time."

I was trying to explain the situation to security when the nurse opened the double doors for the patient's mother to go to the back. Mom made it to the other side, turned around, and motioned for the others to follow her, like she was being slick or something. When she did this, the pregnant girlfriend, the aggressive boy, and two other teens sprinted to the back.

"Hey," the nurse and I both yelled.

"I'm going to kill someone," the raging teen could be heard shouting as he ran down the hallway. He didn't even know which room he was going to. None of them did.

"We'll be down there in just a second," the security guard told me.

But as soon as we hung up, another code was called overhead. Security was needed for a violent patient on the mental health floor. It wasn't going to be 'just a second' before security could make it to the ER. We were on our own.

A minute or two later, the teenagers who'd all run to the back were essentially forced out of the ER by a group of nurses walking side-by-side, forming a human barricade. (Seriously, don't piss off nurses who've not had the chance to pee, eat, or sit down for hours. It doesn't end well.)

One of the nurses looked to me. "Tell security they need to get down here *now*. And Wanda wants the consent form the kid's mom signed. She's trying to get everything ready for the flight team."

I nodded and grabbed the consent form I'd forgotten from the desk as I had security paged again.

"They're busy," the operator said. "Didn't you hear the code a few minutes ago?"

"I mean when they're done," I explained. "I know they're busy, but we have some wild stuff going on down here tonight."

"Yeah," she replied, "it's like that all over this place right now."

We hung up and I looked at the consent form the kid's mom signed. You know, all that time I thought she was signing her name, but all she managed to write was 'mom,' and even that took some effort to decipher.

Wanda came to the desk. "I need that signature sheet."

I shook my head. "I'm making up one that says the patient and adult couldn't sign due to ETOH."

I showed her the form.

She snickered. "Yeah, well we're back there taking bets on which of the two is more hammered: mom or son."

The trouble-making teenagers saw the nurse and ran to the desk.

"Let us back. It's been long enough."

"Oh," the nurse scoffed, "you're not getting back to my ER, not after what you did earlier. I'm sorry, but you're not going to come in here acting this way and get very far."

And that's when the aggressive boy seemed to lose his mind.

He started shoving his friends—including the pregnant girl—and began punching walls. The entire time this was going on, he was either screaming like a banshee or roaring.

I dialed the operator.

"Need security to come here now," I said in a rush.

"I can see if they can call you, but they have this—."

"Need security now," I repeated. "We have a situation."

It didn't take long for the same guard from earlier to return my call.

"What's all that yelling?" he asked.

I quickly explained what was going on and he promised he was on the way.

The teenager was destroying the waiting room, kicking chairs around and turning over tables. His friends were screaming for him to settle down, but I don't know if he could hear them over his own shouts. He walked over to the phone on the waiting room wall and started slamming the receiver against the base of the phone.

And then he started to remove his shirt.

"Get out of here," the pregnant girl yelled, once she saw security approaching. "She called their security guy."

This seemed to spook the teen. He tried sprinting through the waiting room, down the hall, and through the lobby. The entire time, his shirt was stuck over his head, blinding him. He was still throwing punches.

The situation ended when the teenager tried to run from security and ran smack-dab, face-first, into the glass door. He bounced away from the door and landed on his back.

Security showed mercy and didn't call the cops. All of the teenagers were told to leave the hospital property, with the threat that if they returned, local law enforcement would be notified.

The minor patient was flown to another hospital shortly after all of this happened. His mother was arrested for drunk driving a block from the hospital and was brought in for a medical clearance almost as soon as she left. A few weeks later, I encountered the patient's pregnant girlfriend again. She came in with a different boyfriend and was just as *pleasant* to deal with as she was that night.

On the plus side, we didn't have to activate any other traumas that night, and none of the other patients were as unruly as that group.

Pizza Party

Two delivery women from Pizza Hut showed up with 16 small pizzas. This, in itself, isn't odd around here. Families on hospice or OB floors sometimes order tons of food, and sometimes staff from different floors have pizza party nights and all chip in to pay cash. This usually ends well for the delivery people, as they walk away with big tips. The two women told me they needed to get upstairs. I asked if they knew where they were headed, and they said yes, so I simply buzzed them through the locked doors.

Well, shortly after this, I started receiving phone calls from upstairs. The unit clerk up there wanted to know if I could help the pizza girls find someone named 'Mary.'

I couldn't.

Fifteen minutes later, the delivery women came through the ER again. They were both laughing.

And they both still had all 16 pizzas.

"Couldn't find her?" I asked.

"It was a patient," one woman told me.

I shrugged. "So? What's the problem?"

"It was a *mental health* patient," she emphasized. "She said she ordered food for a dinner party."

Apparently, the patient's phone's outside dialing had been activated. Once she figured it out, she made a few calls.

Thankfully, the delivery women weren't too upset about the event.

A female came in because her period was 8 weeks late. When the nurse asked if the patient was sexually active, the female replied she was not.

The pregnancy test determined that was a lie.

When the patient learned she was pregnant, she said she thought the nurse was asking if she was sexually active *now,* and she never thought of the possibility that she could be pregnant because she read online there was something like a 1-in-4 chance of getting pregnant from unprotected sex and, since she and her partner only had sex once, she "should've been okay."

Ask WHY Before Becoming Upset

A mentally disabled man was brought in by a caretaker from his group home. There was a thin line of blood trickling down his face from under a special helmet he wore due to regular falls.

The man's new caretaker pushed his wheelchair to the registration desk and sighed.

"What happened?" I asked.

She shook her head in frustration.

"I told him to stay in bed. I tell him all the time. But what does he do the second I walk away? He gets out of bed and hits his head on a table."

The patient stirred in his chair.

"Just stay sitting," the caretaker scolded him.

She looked at me and rolled her eyes. "He even tried getting up after I found him and put him in his chair. It's like he's hellbent on getting up tonight."

I entered the patient in the system and informed his caretaker that it would only be a minute or so before a nurse could come to the desk for him. I asked both to stay put, rather than waste time trying to get to the waiting room.

During this time, the patient pushed himself out of his wheelchair and held himself up by gripping the registration counter.

I thought the caretaker was going to flip her lid. She turned red, her hands started shaking, and she shouted at the patient, "Stop trying to get up!"

The patient, who'd been in our ER many times before and *never* spoke any of the times he'd been there, looked right at the woman and said in a firm stutter, "I have to pee. Leave me alone."

It turns out, that was the only issue. As soon as the patient was able to relieve himself, he returned to his wheelchair, let the doctor and nurses examine the scratch on his head, and stayed seated the rest of his visit.

Thinking Ahead

We have a frequently-visiting patient who's a little...off. In fact, each time he comes to the ER, one of us has to call the cops for the man's behavior. He once came in, claiming he was poisoned, which is why he broke into his neighbor's apartment—you know, to find the cure.

One morning, as I was impatiently waiting to clock out, the man arrived.

"Great," I muttered to myself as he was walking inside.

A few seconds later, three squad cars pulled up in front of the ER.

Immediately, I figured the guy had already been in trouble that morning and the cops followed him to the hospital.

No.

The man *called the police on his own* and asked them to meet him at the hospital, since it "always ends up this way, anyhow."

No Match for Veruca Salt

A patient was brought in via ambulance on a night I had come in early. Up front, we didn't know a whole lot about what was going on, other than rumors that the patient's car had been hit by a train. Even patients in the waiting room had heard the news and were whispering about it. We expected it to be pretty bad.

The patient, I think, had to be the luckiest teen alive.

This patient just received her license on the day in question. She decided to take her *brand new* Mustang Convertible out for a drive. She said she wanted to 'show off' for her friends, who were following behind her in a not-so-new car.

She lost to the train, and her car was pushed 50 feet down the tracks before the train could come to a complete stop.

Amazingly enough, the patient, who'd been extracted from the car by the local fire department, didn't have much more than a few scratches on her. Her car was totaled and her cell phone was destroyed in the accident.

The patient soon started to get on the nerves of the staff. She complained about her examination, complained that the visit was taking too long, drove nurses out of her room so she could scream at her father and demand another new car, and could be heard shrieking because she didn't have a phone to use to text and update Facebook. She asked for a drink, and when the tech brought her a paper cup filled with ice water, the patient threw the cup against the wall and yelled that she wanted a specific brand of bottled water.

For lack of better or not so crude words, the patient seemed like an ungrateful brat. Even her father became frustrated with her attitude and left the room. Mom swooped in and coddled the girl, telling her everything would be okay and the patient could use her phone until the phone store opened in the morning and they could buy the teen a replacement.

Not too long after the incident, the patient was driving around in her replacement car, another Mustang Convertible, and was arrested for driving under the influence of drugs and alcohol.

Post-Vacation Blues

A female patient was brought in via ambulance for chest pain. At least 20 of her family members flooded the lobby, demanding to hear updates and to be let to the back to visit her. I explained to the family that there was often a waiting period for nurses and doctors to examine patients and run necessary tests, so they could have a seat in the waiting room and someone would allow them back two at a time to visit with the patient when the time was right.

And, surprisingly, none of the members argued with me about this. Everyone sat down, except for an older man: the patient's father. He approached the desk and said sternly to me, "Nobody is to know she's here."

"If I mark her 'no' to our hospital directory," I explained, "at no time can I acknowledge she is here. So that means, you know, I recognize you, and I can make an exception for you, but if someone else from your family comes to the desk—from the waiting room or from outside—I have to say I don't have her listed as a patient."

"That's fine," he said with a nod. "I also need you to remove her husband from her emergency contact list. He has absolutely no business in her life after what happened tonight."

The patient's father didn't elaborate. I confirmed these changes with the patient via her nurse a few minutes later, and everything was fine.

Dad, every now and then, escorted one other family member back to see the patient.

Then, all of the sudden, things somehow got out of hand. I was taking a phone call and dad came to the desk again, this time with two people.

I covered the phone's mouthpiece and explained only two visitors could go back at a time.

"I'll send someone out," he stated.

He didn't send anyone out. I learned that when the patient's nurse called me to the back and wanted to know why I let eight visitors back at the same time.

The visitors fled. Some left for a while.

And then they came back, at least six of them, all toting boxes and suitcases and rolling luggage filled with personal belongings.

"We need to leave these with you," one of the patient's family members said to me.

I shook my head. "I can't be responsible for personal effects."

"It's not going to be for long," the man tried to reason. "Her husband should be here soon to pick it up. He's not to see her. You're just going to give him his stuff and tell him to find another place to live."

I scoffed. "I'm not getting in the middle of family drama. You'll have to take care of this yourself."

"It's not like we're asking you to file divorce papers for them," he argued.

"I am *not* getting involved in this," I repeated firmly.

The man was mad.

"She won't do it," he announced to his family.

Just about this time, the patient's husband pulled up outside the ER and parked his SUV. He was shouting as he made his way inside, and the women from the patient's family were trying to corral the men, acting as barriers to keep their husbands from fighting with the patient's husband.

Security saw the scuffle and came out of their office. The argument died down and the patient's husband loaded his belongings in his vehicle. He continued to shout and curse, but he eventually left.

Very soon after, we all learned (from family members telling us all about it) the patient and her family had returned from the Bahamas that morning. Everything was fine, or so it seemed. But then the patient's young son pulled her aside and told her that his step-father had molested him. The patient, experiencing the full spectrum of emotions, went outside to catch her breath. She passed out and hit her head on her concrete landscaping bricks. When she came to, she thought she was having a heart attack, so her kids called 911. Her husband thought he was going to be arrested, so he bolted. While the patient was in the ER, her family went to her house, packed up all the husband's things, and changed the locks.

<u>People Are Strange...</u>

It's no secret we get a few weirdos around this place. Here are a few we've had just hanging around:

-About every two days, at 2 a.m., a man leans his bicycle up against the hospital's exterior, comes inside, asks if he can use the bathroom, and then he stays in there about 20 minutes. Each time he leaves, he politely gives us a warning: "I pooped, so you should stay out of there for a while."

-I once called security after I noticed a man walking around near the ER entrance. That part wasn't a huge deal, but the fact that I'd noticed him outside three hours in a row did raise a red flag. Security asked the man if he was visiting or needed medical treatment. He said he lived across the street but couldn't go back to his apartment because it was haunted.

-Around 3 a.m., security questioned a man who'd been sitting on the sidewalk outside the ER door. He showed them that his hands were full of white powdered doughnuts, and he said he had to stay there until it stopped raining so his doughnuts wouldn't get wet.

-I was walking to my car at 4 in the morning and noticed a man seemed to show up out of nowhere and was watching me, but when I would glance over at him, he'd turn away. As soon as I went back inside, I told security about the incident. They searched the parking lot, but the man was gone. An hour later, they found him in another one of the hospital's lots. He was lying on the ground, waving his hands over his face. Security approached the man, who asked, "Am I dead? Did I die and go to Hell? It's so dark here." We're fairly certain some pretty strong drugs were involved in this.

Priorities

A female was brought in via ambulance for taking bath salts. At first she was unresponsive, but she came to rather quickly and went crazy. She pulled her jeans down to her ankles, got her handcuffed wrists stuck around her knees, and the cop at her bedside had to uncuff her just to help her get loose. The patient then started screaming and accusing everyone around her of being involved in a satanic cult, and she swore her purpose in life was to kill all the cult members.

In the middle of this meltdown, the patient stopped her screaming, seemed sad, and asked, "Does this mean they're going to take away my kids?"

The cop answered, "Well, you *did* overdose and leave your baby in the kitchen sink, so probably. What do you think happens when your six-year-old has to call 911 because mommy is sleeping on the floor?"

And, no kidding, the patient started to cry and said, "So I'll lose my child support, too?"

A young father brought in a toddler who'd been crying because his feet hurt. Dad said they'd gone to the zoo that day and the toddler wanted to walk for the most part, but he'd stopped to cry several times, and now dad just thought it was the right time to bring the boy to be seen.

It didn't take too long to figure out what was wrong.

The patient had been wearing his sneakers on the wrong feet all day.

No Words

So, every now and then, a patient presents with something I can't handle. That something is always vomit. Through my own gags, I rapidly explain to the patient someone else will see him/her in a moment, and I also explain I have to step away.

The only other time I had to hand off a patient registration was when I was laughing so hard I couldn't see through my tears.

A teen patient and her boyfriend came to the desk to register for something that had happened to them during intercourse.

According to the patient, things were going well in bed...until she 'farted from the vagina.' This scared the patient and her boyfriend so much they decided to come to the ER at almost midnight so they could have her checked out.

My coworker finished registering the patient and a doctor explained to the young couple that this is a "completely natural" occurrence.

I've lost count of how many patients have returned just a few hours after being diagnosed with the flu, a cold, broken bones, or food poisoning because they were still sick or still felt pain. All of them were under the impression that simply receiving a diagnosis would help them heal faster, I suppose. Triage has had to explain to some of them that they actually have to *take* the prescribed medication to feel better, not just have the prescription filled.

Thirsty

One evening, shortly before visiting hours ended, the operator announced a fire in the building. When a fire alarm code is called, some doors automatically release from their open positions and lock closed, while staff members are responsible for closing all other doors.

I had just closed the triage door when I noticed a woman trying to get through the double doors at the end of the hall.

Over the repetitive fire alarm, I called to the woman, "You can't go through there right now."

I pointed to the flashing emergency lights on the hall wall and said, "A fire has been announced."

The woman, who'd been waiting in the waiting room to be seen because her blood sugar was too high, became angry.

"I'm thirsty," she said.

I shrugged and said politely, "Sorry, but I can't open any of the doors until an all clear is announced."

The patient punched the door and screamed, "I just want a freakin' Mountain Dew!"

So, not only was she seen for her high blood sugar, but she also was seen for the two fingers she broke when she hit the door.

Dad brought in daughter because her skin was 'on-fire red,' and he was certain she was allergic to the shirt mom bought for the girl that morning.

She wasn't allergic. The girl had worked up a sweat during the day, causing the shirt's dye to bleed, leaving red ink on the girl's upper region.

An average-sized, retired family doctor was asked to step on the scale during the triage process, but he became belligerent and refused.

The triage nurse explained to the M.D. that it was vital to know the patient's weight to work up a chart, but the patient still refused.

He kicked the scale and left, only to return a few hours later because he was 'pretty sure' he'd broken his big toe when he unleashed his frustrations on the scale.

The kicker to all of this was the patient had to get on the scale to complete the triage process and be seen for his toe injury.

"You don't have to talk to me like a normal person," I overheard a patient say to the doctor as I stood in the hall and waited for my chance to complete his registration.

"I've been studying medicine for a while now, and I understand how you sometimes just want to be able to talk to an equal."

The doctor actually sounded pleased when he asked, "Oh, you're in medical school?"

When the patient replied, no, he wasn't in medical school, but he 'really enjoyed' watching shows like *Grey's Anatomy* and *House*, a nurse who'd overheard it and I about died laughing. The doctor left the room and rolled his eyes.

At Least He Didn't Use a Rock and Ice Skate

A patient came in, with a chief complaint of 'dental pain,' but how he explained what was going on wasn't as tactful as simply typing 'dental pain.'

As usual, as I was registering the patient, he told me the tooth had been hurting for several days, but at 2 a.m., he just couldn't take it anymore.

Instead of driving straight to the ER, the patient decided he would head out to the garage first and find some pliers. The patient tried to extract his tooth, but the pliers slipped and he stabbed himself in the lower gums with the tool's handle.

The triage nurse asked the man to open his mouth. When he did, she gasped and said loudly, "Oh my."

That's how I knew it was worse than the patient was letting on.

The patient half-succeeded in extracting his tooth. It was hanging by the tip, but when he stabbed himself with the pliers, he gave up and decided he needed professional help.

His tooth was fully extracted, and he received eight sutures to patch up his torn gums.

106

Guy came in for a medical clearance and two dog bites that required a total of 36 stitches.

When the cops have two canine units holding you and they tell you not to move, thinking you can run before the dogs will leap probably isn't a good idea.

Awkkkkkkwaaaaaard!

A female checked in for abdominal pain and vomiting.

I decided to do a full register at the front desk, just because the lobby was empty and it would be easier than fighting with lab and CT and all the other departments trying to get to the patient when she was in her room.

The patient gave me all of her information and told me she'd gotten married since the last time she'd been in our ER. She wanted her mother bumped down to secondary emergency contact, and she gave me her husband's information so I could list him as primary.

None of this seems abnormal, right?

The patient told me she'd left her house in a hurry and must have forgotten her cell phone, so she asked me if I could call her husband. I guess he went over to a friend's house for a poker game, and she just wanted to let him know she was in the hospital.

Again, no big deal.

Triage took the patient straight back and I made the call to her husband.

The man on the other line sounded groggy.

I gave him my name, told him where I was calling from, and I explained that his wife was in our ER.

He angrily said, "That woman is *not* my wife. She was a customer where I worked, and she began stalking me. I quit my job, changed my home phone number...My wife and I even considered moving. Look, I don't know how she got this number, and I'm sorry you have to get involved in this, but please let everyone there know I already have a wife and that woman is crazy."

So, after I apologized for waking up a stranger at 3:30 in the morning, I went to the back and explained what had just happened.

I guess the people in back found it was more acceptable to just leave well enough alone and treat the patient for what she'd presented, rather than call in a mental health counselor.

A few months later, we did end up reading in the local paper that the patient was arrested for violating an order of protection.

<u>Bath Salts...Not Just for Relaxing</u>

I'd been at work for about 30 seconds before a woman basically dragged herself to the registration desk and puked all over the counter and floor.

The triage nurse, about to call another patient, stopped what she was doing and helped the woman into a wheelchair.

"I took bath salts," the patient screamed. "I need you to get it out of me."

Our triage nurse tried to explain, "There's nothing we can really do to flush it out of your system. The only thing we can really do for you is monitor your vitals. What do you want us to do for you right now?"

"Kill me," the woman shrieked. "Kill me now. I deserve to die for what I've done."

"What did you do?" security asked, coming from around the corner.

"I killed someone tonight. I gave him salts and he's dead, and I did something bad."

Well, that's a good way to get the cops called, let me just say that for those who didn't have an idea.

We registered the patient and she was taken back to a room. She screamed about a 'bad batch' of salts the whole time, but I have to say, as opposed to people saying they had a good time smoking pot and having the munchies or taking 'shrooms and hallucinating, I have *never* heard anyone tell a good story about bath salts. So, maybe I'm wrong, but as she was shouting, I was thinking there was no such thing as a 'good batch' of the stuff.

About every 15 minutes, someone else would come in with the same chief complaint. This happened until we had six rooms with bath salt users. It was almost impossible to walk through the back part of the ER without hearing people gagging and barfing, screaming, crying, apologizing, cursing...It was a madhouse. I took paperwork back and was walking back to the front when I saw one of the users violently jerk forward from a lying position, and he then projectile vomited all over the floor and counter that was about two feet away. His primary nurse was taking it rather well, if 'rather well' means screeching, "I told you to use the bag!"

Then the police showed up...As in, there were seven squad cars parked outside the ER entrance and at least 11 officers patrolling the lobby and back ER, not including the hospital's own security department. These cops wanted to know everything there was to know about the patients and what had happened to lead them all to the ER.

While they were interviewing the patients, a tall, almost-toothless man came to the desk.

"My wife's here," he said.

"And who's your wife?" I asked.

He gave me the name of the first bath salts woman.

Well, everyone in the ER—including other people waiting, either to be seen or to visit current patients—knew the cops were looking for this man. He must have known it, too, because he nervously glanced around, looked to me, and said, "You know, never mind."

As soon as he turned to leave, I headed to the back to let the cops know their guy was walking out the door.

A female cop took off running, and it was a good thing, too, because the man was also sprinting across the parking lot.

We all watched on the security monitors as the cop raced across the lot, jumped in the air, and took the fleeing man down with a hard tackle that would put any pro football player to shame.

The patient's husband was arrested for another drug-related crime, but he did repeat the story about someone dying from taking bath salts that night...He just didn't know where his friends dumped the body, and he said he doubted they knew, either, because they were all in the ER battling 107-degree fevers, seizures, tachycardia, and loss of consciousness.

To my knowledge, a body was never found. We kind of theorized that the patients had hallucinated that part, but I guess we'll never be positive unless they gave the cops the name of a person and that person was verified as being alive.

All I really know is, unfortunately, this was not our first experience with bath salts, and I highly doubt it will be the last.

Dad brought in a newborn with a wound to the leg. He was left alone with the baby for the first time, after arguing with his wife about his capability to do so without something bad happening. I'd say it was going *real well*, considering he was in the ER at midnight.

His wife had been gone an hour when he decided to vacuum as the baby was lying on a play mat on the floor. He said he was distracted by something on TV and accidentally ran the baby's leg over with the vacuum. The baby's skin was puckered, red, and torn in a small spot.

The doctor used glue to close the wound. No word on dad after that night.

Once had a mom bring in her teen because they went to the movies and he ate some popcorn he dropped on the seat. He said it tasted funny, so he used his cell phone to look at the seat and noticed there was blood on the fabric, so he and mom wanted an immediate HIV test, just in case he was infected from the popcorn he ate 15 minutes ago.

Believe it or not, out of all the stories I have, this is one everyone thinks is fake, but the kid sat on the bench and sobbed the entire time his mom was talking because he was scared he was going to die.

A Sew-Dire Dental Emergency

A college girl came to the desk at two in the morning and pointed back to her friend.

"She needs to be seen by a doctor," the girl told me.

"What's going on with her?" I asked. I tried to look over to the patient, but she was sitting on the bench, freaking out, and was surrounded by her friends.

"She has something stuck in her teeth."

"Something stuck in her teeth? Like food?"

"No."

The patient was trying to get popcorn remnants out from between her teeth and decided to use a sewing needle to do this. She stuck the needle between her two front teeth and couldn't get it out. The girl was scared to death she was going to lose her teeth if she tried to jerk it out.

I guess her nurse just wiggled the needle every which direction until it came loose.

The patient was sent home with discharge instructions that recommended using floss.

<u>And?</u>

An older gentleman came in for a wheelchair shortly before my coworker clocked out. Several minutes later, he wheeled his wife to the registration desk.

"What brings you here tonight?" I asked.

They both stared at me for 15 seconds, as if I was supposed to already know. A lot of people actually do this. I repeated my question.

The woman's husband snapped to me, "Well, it's her time of the month."

I looked to the 50+ year-old and kind of hoped she'd help me along so I could enter the complaint. She didn't, so I looked back to the husband. "And she's just here tonight for menstrual problems?"

"Well did I say she was?" he asked in a raised voice.

So, I asked my original question. "What brings you here tonight?"

"I was here a few months ago, about six months, for a fall," the woman said.

Sometimes I want to shake people and say, "Tell me what's wrong **tonight**."

"Okay..." I stated.

"Well?" the husband asked. "Why aren't you typing anything? Why aren't you getting a doctor to see her?"

My coworker took a deep breath but kept to himself.

"I'm a little at loss for what's going on right now."

"We already told you two things," the woman said, annoyed. "I don't know what's so hard about this. Maybe if they'd get some better help in here..."

My coworker laughed, that exasperated kind of chuckle that comes out when you just really can't take anymore BS.

"So," he asked, "you're here because you're on your period and you fell six months ago? Is that why you're here?"

The woman's husband sighed and said loudly, dragging out the 'o' in his response, "No. I brought her here tonight because she fell in the kitchen about an hour ago and needs to be checked out. I don't know how you two have jobs."

I don't know what the lady's period and a fall all that time ago had to do with each other, but I am still kind of curious to know how the patient and her husband think they correlate.

The patient was taken to the back. Her complaint was changed on the tracking board to 'abd pain,' 'nausea,' and 'muscle spasms,' before someone finally settled on 'multiple complaints.'

Put You Right to Sleep

At seven in the morning, a patient was wheeled to the desk by his wife.

"What seems to be the problem this morning?" I asked.

His wife shrugged. "I can't even tell you because I don't know."

"Ballpark it for me," I suggested. "We just need to have a general idea."

The wife looked confused. "What does that mean?"

I smiled politely. "Is he vomiting? Is he in pain? Did he fall?"

She shook her head. "No. He just won't sleep."

The patient cleared his throat to catch his wife's attention. She looked at him, widened her eyes, and looked back at me.

"Oh," she said, "and he's in a lot of pain."

"Okay."

I entered the patient in the system and only then learned from his wife that he'd been discharged from the ER at 11 the night before...which was right when I was clocking in.

Okay, oh well, no big deal. This isn't something uncommon.

Fifteen minutes after the patient was taken

back to a room, he came walking out to the lobby, somehow miraculously cured of his inability to walk in in the first place. His wife was shaking her head and the patient was shaking a fistful of papers.

He turned to me and shouted, "And let me tell you something, Missy. The doctor back there right now is a jackass. He's rude and has absolutely no business practicing medicine because he doesn't really care about people."

This was the same doctor who often saw employees free of charge and would go out of his way to say hello to everyone around him, the same doctor who'd buy the entire ER and visiting departments (Respiratory, CT, X-Ray) pizza just for the heck of it.

But he was also the one you could always count on to get tired real quick of some of the frequent complaints.

According to the patient's wife, her husband wanted another dose of Dilaudid and more pills, because the two 'lost' the first 2-week dose the patient had been prescribed a few hours earlier. The patient, I guess, then told the doctor he couldn't sleep, to which the doctor responded, "Of course you can't sleep; you were asleep the whole time you were here last night. It's not insomnia, it's called a sleeping rhythm."

The patient's wife said the doctor declared another dose of Dilaudid would *not* be administered, nor would he write another prescription for the 'lost' pills.

Grandma and mom brought in a toddler with a fever.

Triage took the child's temperature.

106.8 degrees, the highest temp registered in our ER, according to the nurses in back.

When asked when the child's last dose of medicine was, grandma and mom said they didn't believe in giving the child medicine. The kid had the fever for three hours before someone at church recommended they bring her in to be seen.

The baby was transferred to a pediatric hospital due to a life-threatening condition that was causing her fever.

<u>Waiting His Turn</u>

The lobby was full of people needing to be seen, mostly for things like congestion or headaches or coughing. I noticed an older man, probably in his late 80s, sit on the bench and patiently wait for the line to get shorter.

Finally, after about six minutes, it was his turn.

The elderly man came to the desk and said to me, with his hand across his heart, "It feels like there's a small cat sitting on my chest."

Once we got him situated in a wheelchair and called the back for someone to take him to a room and start tests, I asked him why he chose a cat, as opposed to the animals we usually hear, and I definitely wanted to know why he waited when he was having chest pains.

This man was so sweet and so kind he shook his head and said, "Dear, I don't believe in exaggerating my condition when there are sure to be other people in here who need help more than I do, and my mamma and daddy always taught me to wait my turn."

It turns out the man was having a heart attack and was sent off to Cath Lab. We didn't have the chance to speak again because his procedure didn't go as well as planned, and he passed away an hour after arriving on the ICU.

These Are the People I Deal With

I was having one of those nights when I couldn't get anything done. The waiting room was packed and the back was full. Wait times were anywhere from 30 to 90 minutes, depending on these rushes that would come and go of seriously ill patients versus people coming in with complaints of runny noses.

Finally, as it was dying down, a woman stormed up to the desk and demanded to know why they hadn't called her up to be seen.

I asked the patient's name, but she wasn't on the board to be seen. She was livid.

"Did someone else check you in?" I asked.

She shook her head and told me, no, I was the only one at the desk when she had come in.

Well, I knew I didn't register the woman, and I told her such, that she wasn't registered in the system.

"Well, I *know* that," she said bitterly. "I have been in the waiting room for an hour, wondering when you were going to come and get my information."

The woman was dead serious and I know it's wrong, but I wanted to slap her with my clipboard. I signed her in for something like dental pain or a cold sore. And...surprise! She left before being seen because "the wait was too long."

ETOH patient called for an ambulance because he thought he was dead.

Logic...

BAC was .38-something.

Had a new (hysterical) mom bring in her two-week-old baby because he wouldn't stop crying and he hadn't had a wet diaper for some time. Baby also had a fever for a few days.

Quickly found out mom followed grandma's advice of 'feed a cold, starve a fever' a bit too literally and hadn't fed the baby in *two days*, hence the crying, I'm sure.

A nurse fed the baby a bottle and he went straight to sleep. CPS was called to talk to the new (and highly-embarrassed) mom.

Hmmm...

I was walking outside to take a break when I saw an ambulance pull in. Knowing the EMT would need a face sheet, I cursed a bit and went back inside.

The EMT was cursing more than I had when he came to the desk.

"What's wrong?" I asked.

"These people take advantage of our services when there are other people out there, you know, dying," he grunted.

I was confused, but figured the patient's diagnosis was something trivial.

And it was. 'Nose pain.'

The ambulance service left and the patient was discharged within 30 minutes.

After nurses released the patient to the waiting room, he practically ran to the phone in the waiting room and furiously dialed.

"I can't get this phone to work," he shouted to me.

I instructed the patient he had to dial a number to reach an outside line, but he still couldn't figure it out, so I had to help him dial his friend's number.

And then he told me, I swear, "I ran out of minutes on my cell phone, and this is the only place I know that has a free phone to use, so I came here to call my friends."

<u>Whole Life Story</u>

I had an elderly man come to the desk this morning. His lips, cheeks, eyelids, and hands were swollen.

"Should I be seen for this?" he asked.

I told the man I couldn't offer medical advice, but *I* would definitely want to be seen if I experienced the kind of swelling he was.

"Did you get stung by a bee or eat something new that you could be allergic to?" I asked, thinking the man could narrow it down.

"Well," he thought aloud. "See, yesterday I went over to my friend's house. She's actually a little more than a friend, but we don't want our families knowing that because they'll cause all sorts of ruckus about it."

I tried to interject, but he was talking a mile a minute, and I hate interrupting people.

"So, you see, I helped her pull some weeds. And then she asked if I was hungry—and I was—so she wanted to drive to Cincinnati, but I wanted to stay local. But when you love someone, you just do what they want to do, so over to Cincinnati we went."

He continued, "Now, we usually take the highway, but part of it was closed, so we had to go through this little town. And we stopped because she wanted to browse through an antique shop. But most of what they had in there was pure junk, I'm tellin' you. So, after about an hour of browsing, she finally settled on this cast iron skillet. I told her I had one she could have, no use wastin' her money on something I could give her free. So she put it back on the shelf and we took off again. Got to Cincinnati about three."

Oh my gosh, I thought to myself. *It's never going to end, is it?*

"Well, we don't get to Cincinnati but maybe once a month. Like to save those trips for date nights. We've been going to the city for about, I don't know...Eight years I think I've been seeing her, but only five if you count it being appropriate, as her husband was alive for the first three. And, well, we like to go to this nice restaurant on the east side of town, but this time we went to the one on the west side."

I opened my mouth to speak, but he kept going.

"See, the restaurants are owned by the same people and are even named the same thing, but the food doesn't taste the same because they have different cooks working at both. But, generally, the menu is the same. I prefer the place on the east side. I could definitely tell the difference. If you blindfolded me and let me taste their chicken Parmesan, I could tell you which one of their restaurants it came from, I guarantee it."

Finally, the man took a breath and I was able

to fully register him.

I guess he was able to finish telling the rest of his story, like the part where he had a minor allergy to strawberries and 'maybe that's why that pie was red.'

And This is How You Make Everyone Hate You

I planned on getting a little bit of extra sleep that night, but my coworkers called me three times in a row, so I figured I'd probably better get up and find out what they needed so badly.

They needed help.

The parking lot was full when I pulled in, and I ended up parking 10 light years away, just to walk by five cop cars and push my way through the crowded lobby of people giving me dirty looks.

"You're not cutting in front of me," growled one man to me. "I've been waiting in this line for 15 minutes and I think I'm dying."

"I work here," I responded. "And I doubt you're dying, so give me a minute to clock in and we'll try to get this line moving."

The girl up front was overwhelmed, almost to the point of crying.

"These floors keep calling, yelling at me," she said in a broken voice. "And people are coming in left and right. I don't know what to do."

She said our other coworker was in the back, trying desperately to green the full tracking board.

OB called to ask why the new baby they called down 20 minutes ago wasn't in the system, and then ICU wanted to know what was taking so long on a bed transfer. Within two minutes of being there, I answered seven calls like that.

"What is taking so long?" a woman approaching the desk asked in a snippy and loud voice. "This is the emergency department, right?"

"Sure is," I answered. "Are you having one right now?"

"My son can't breathe through one of his nostrils. We need to get him checked in."

I glanced to the 12-year-old and then back to the mom.

That was sure some emergency, by golly.

I told my coworker to hand me all the paperwork from her floor calls and to focus only on the people in front of her. I sped through chart after chart, and about five minutes later, I had made all the necessary changes and stepped up to help my coworker.

Half of the people in the lobby were sent to the waiting room, but more kept flooding in, and they were all convinced they were high priority, with cold and flu symptoms, congestion, headaches, and diarrhea.

But then a chest pain came in, and the patient was loud about it.

We put him in the wheelchair and he screamed and screamed that we needed to get him to the back. The triage nurse came out of her room and asked the patient multiple questions before deciding to try to find him a bed. Several other people in the lobby were groaning and moaning.

"Maybe I should have chest pain, too," a woman curtly said to someone behind her.

'I've had it from the second I walked in the door,' I thought to myself.

The chest pain patient wasn't in the back very long. As soon as nurses took the man's shirt off, they put him back in the wheelchair and sent him to the waiting room to go through the triage process. Now, I don't know, exactly, if it was revenge or what, but the man sat in triage and watched five people who'd come in *after* he did get taken back, triaged, and placed in a bed. I wanted to say it was simply based on other diagnoses, but I saw a patient with a jammed finger go back and another with what appeared to be a paper cut get taken back before the man's name was finally called in a tired tone. I did briefly wonder why he was sent back out, but we were all too busy to talk about it.

His chest pain was more external than anything else. I guess he tried waxing for the first time that afternoon and some of his skin came off with his body hair. He had minor scrapes, if that's what you call them, and he said his skin was on fire.

The doctor said it looked like the patient had a minor allergy to the wax, told him the area would heal, and advised him not to do it again.

There's a Time to Come to the ER

Around 3 in the morning on the first night after a holiday weekend, a man brought his wife in to be seen. She was speaking gibberish and the patient's husband said she'd been doing that for two days. She was also experiencing paralysis of her left side, and she was taken straight back.

The patient's husband said the doctor offices around the area were closed for the weekend and holiday, and then they couldn't get an appointment for that morning, so they were going to try to wait until her scheduled appointment—which was two days away. They just 'didn't think' it was 'that serious.'

In actuality, the patient had been having a series of strokes. She was admitted to ICU and stayed a few days.

Do it Yourself

A teenager came to the registration desk with his mom, but before I could start the registration process, the teen became angry and walked out. His mom was shouting at him as they left the building, and I could see on the security monitors that the two were arguing directly outside the ER. This happens from time to time, especially with mental health cases, so I didn't give it much thought.

Minutes later, mom and son returned to the desk.

"What seems to be the problem tonight?" I asked.

The teen boy lifted the sleeve of his shirt to show me a huge bump on his inner forearm. It was oozing from between scabbing and it smelled. The skin around the edges was turning black.

"He's been hiding this from me," his mom said, "because he hates going to the doctor."

"Is it a bite or...?" I asked.

The thing was probably just a tad bit smaller than the top of a coke can.

"I think it's a spider bite," mom said. "We were cleaning out the garage about a week and a half ago, and we had to have an exterminator come out and get rid of some recluses."

I nodded.

"But he hid it," mom said, "and then I found out he's been lancing it himself and trying to clean it out with Pine Sol."

The patient admitted to doing this five times since he was bitten. Instead of helping the wound heal, the combination of the self-lancing and the spider bite resulted in a nasty infection. Switchboard called and said they could all hear the boy scream when the doctors had to open the wound and clean it out.

Bloody ~~Patience~~ Patients

Triage had an *interesting* patient one night. The young girl was fairly grumpy with me at the registration desk, when she was checking in for abdominal cramping, but she took took her attitude to a whole-new-level as soon as she got back with the nurse.

To every question the triage nurse asked, the patient's response was, "And why do you need to know that?"

Triage explained several nurses were likely to ask the same questions multiple times to take in account the patient's medical history and to stay on top of information in order to treat her pain, which, of course, the patient said was a 10/10...as she sipped from a Big Gulp and kept texting her friends, despite the nurse's polite request that she not do either at the moment.

"And when was your last menstrual cycle?" asked the nurse.

"My what?"

"Menstrual cycle."

"I don't know what that is. Are you doing this on purpose? Are you wasting my time on purpose?"

"Your period," the nurse broke it down. "When was your last period?"

The patient laughed. "Right now."

"So you're on your period right now?"

"That's what I just said, isn't it?"

There was a pause. "Do you think your abdominal and pelvic cramping could just be your period?"

Her male friend, sitting right next to her in triage, added, "If you're gonna be talking about this kind of stuff, I can't be around. I just can't."

He tried to get out of triage, but the patient bit his head off. He was sweating and looked like he was going to vomit or pass out or both, as he was caught between the triage room and the registration area. He was desperate to get out of there, but it was clear his friend ran all operations.

"Well," triage said to the man, "you can go back out to the waiting room. We're going to have to perform a gynecological exam, and this is just the best for patient privacy. When we're through, we can send someone out to bring you back."

He breathed a sigh of relief.

"Uh, no," the patient yelled loudly. "He's not allowed to leave. He *told me* he was coming to the hospital with me, and he's going to be with me."

He begged with a whine, "Please don't make me do this. I can't do this."

Triage stepped in again and told the patient the room was too small to have her friend back, that too many doctors and nurses would be occupying the space.

The patient's friend went to sit down, and she

141

was taken back to an exam room.

Nobody ever came to get the friend, mostly, I think, because the patient wasn't in the room very long. She was given a heating pad to use over her lower abdomen during her visit, and the nurse gave her some $320 Tylenol. The girl's pain went away within a half hour, leading the girl's formal diagnosis to be 'Menstrual Cycle.'

I was walking a few things to the back when the patient came out of her room and shook papers in my face. When I say 'in my face,' I don't mean that she was standing two feet away, shaking papers in the air. No, the edges of two papers scraped the tip of my nose.

"Go get my nurse, and get her fast," she barked.

"I saw you're discharged," I said politely, trying to help the situation. The back was getting busy, and when I have to track nurses down, they always want to know if I tried to remedy the situation first, and then they want to know details of the patient's concern. "Are you confused about your instructions?"

She nodded and laughed. "Yes, I am, because I don't have this."

She pointed to some of the things that could accompany a period.

"See?" she said, pointing to the words, 'bloating, tenderness, high or low emotions, hunger.' "I don't have half of these. You people have no idea what you're doing."

"These are just general symptoms that go along with this diagnosis," I tried to explain. I knew the girl's nurse was busy, trying to get another patient ready for a transfer to ICU. "This doesn't mean you'll have every last one of these things; it just means this could be part of it."

"Are you a nurse? Do you have the 'RN' badge under your name?" she asked condescendingly.

"No, but—."

I wanted to tell her, 'but I have common sense.'

"You're arguing with a customer right now," she told me gruffly. "People like me keep you with a job. *(I didn't say anything at the time, but isn't that the damn truth?!)* You know my Medicaid pays you, right?"

A lot of people in our hospital worry about Press Ganey scores.

I'm not generally one of them. I probably should be, but I'm mostly a 'treat people the way you want to be treated, unless you really can't take it anymore, and then maybe treating people the way they treat you isn't so bad every now and again' kind of person.

"I'm pretty sure that's the other way around," I told the girl. "But if you really need to see a *nurse* to tell you the same thing I just told you, I'll be sure to go get one."

"Good," she snorted, sticking her nose in the air.

I had to interrupt the patient's nurse, just as she was preparing her unresponsive trauma patient's oxygen tank for transport.

"Your period-patient wants you," I told her.

She cussed. "I knew she was going to be trouble from the second she opened her mouth. She did nothing but berate me the whole time I was in there. She told me she couldn't trust a fat nurse, and when I told her I was *pregnant,* she still had something to say."

The nurse thought for a second and told me to go find the no-nonsense doctor. He didn't treat the girl, but the nurse thought maybe he should have to avoid all of the trouble she gave everyone who'd been involved with her visit to the ER.

I tracked down the doctor and told him about the patient, as well as made sure to add the nurse specifically requested his assistance.

I didn't hear all of what the doctor told the patient, but she tried one last time, as he was trying to move her toward the exit, to argue with the discharge instructions.

"Just keep them around," he smiled. "Unless you get pregnant, you'll have one again next month and we'd hate it if you had to single-handedly keep this place open because you're bloated. Those instructions will explain everything."

<u>Speaking of Those Pesky Press Ganey Surveys...</u>

Our department gets scolded for poor scores. Most negative scores include statements like this:

"They didn't offer me anything to eat."

or

"They made me wait for 20 minutes because the machine in the next room was beeping fast."

or

"They gave me enough pills to make it through the night, but then told me to see my primary doctor. Why do I need one if you're open all night?"

or

"She told me it'd take a second to register me because there was a 'life or death' case she had to deal with. How did she know my cough wasn't life or death?"

So we've all been talking about this and think it should be perfectly acceptable to send the patient

145

a post card with that *Hangover* meme: "But did you die?"

A patient came to the desk at three in the morning to register for abdominal pain. She said she and her husband were leaving for Jamaica at in a few hours, but she just wanted to have it checked out and possibly get medication, if needed.

The patient's appendix was on the verge of bursting, so she was told she was being transferred to surgery.

This did not make her happy.

"I just wanted them to tell me what was wrong and give me a pill to take," she grumbled to me, as I finished her bedside registration. "But now they've gone off and ruined my trip."

A man came in because the floor in his 'new' early-1900s house gave way. Kid you not...he put a ladder up in his kitchen so he could start renovating, some kind of beam gave out, and he ended up in his basement.

"Do you live in a safe environment?" triage asked.

The man's husband thought this was the funniest thing in the world and laughed until he cried.

"Obviously not," said the patient.

The Latest Buzz

It was a pretty slow night and we only had one patient on the board. Granted, he was a frequent flier with mental health issues and occasional violent tendencies, but that night he was behaving himself, or so I thought.

In the dead of night, I heard several of the ER nurses shrieking.

Of course, the first thing on my mind was a video I once saw on CNN, where a man was chasing nurses and doctors around the ER with a pipe or piece of bed railing or something. Maybe something like this is unlikely to happen in any ER and slightly less likely to happen at *this* ER, but I think we've all had concerns of violent patients from time to time.

So, when one of the security guards took off running to the back, I can't say I was feeling all that easy about the situation.

"Oh, you're kidding me!" I heard the man shout.

He came back to the front about a minute later, shaking his head.

"Problems with that guy?" I asked.

He sighed. "A bug. They were all freaking out over a beetle that probably flew right through the front door."

Frequent flier: I was reading WebMd, and when I put in all my symptoms, it said I have a brain tumor and should be checked out in the Emergency Room.

Another patient: You're lucky, then, because whenever I put in my symptoms, it comes back and tells me I have cancer with a 1% survival rate.

Tell Me Sweet Little Lies

22:03-PT presents w back pain x3 days. PT states he was helping a friend move a refrigerator and he felt something pinch. Pain 10/10.

22:33-This RN explains to PT that he must have a ride home to receive rqstd double dosage of Dilaudid. PT states he drove but wife will pick him up after dc.

22:40-Reg dosage x2 administered.

22:55-PT states pain is now 5/10. Pain goal reached. PT again states he will not drive home.

23:00-PT states to doctor wife will drive home. PT restates he will not drive.

23:40-Notified of wife in WR. Confirmed visually. PT dc. PT and wife state PT will not drive. PT warned against driving and possibility of arrest if caught driving. PT enters wife's vehicle.

23:45-PT seen exiting wife's vehicle and driving personal vehicle from parking lot. Doc notified. Local authorities notified.

There is absolutely NO reason to be ashamed of coming to the ER desk if you are serious about quitting drugs and/or alcohol.

I don't have enough fingers and toes to count how many patients have presented to the desk, only to become embarrassed and leave. ALL of the patients I've seen come in for drug and/or alcohol abuse have expressed guilt/shame/embarrassment/nervousness. Some have said they feel like they will be judged by hospital staff. Most say they can't believe the problem has gotten as far as it has.

I've seen teens come in. I've seen men and women in their 70s come in.

It is <u>never</u> too late to get help.

And if you have to check in at 3 p.m. or 3 a.m. to do this, good for you for taking the first step to sobriety and happiness.

True Panic

A group of frat guys came to the desk. One of the man's hands was wrapped in a tee-shirt. He was sweaty and panting. Another guy was holding a Styrofoam cooler. Half of the guys weren't wearing shirts. I think they were all red from being in the sun all day.

"I couldn't come to the party, so you brought the party to me," I joked.

One of the guys stepped forward and pulled the lid off the cooler. He reached in carefully, grabbed something, and rested his forearms on the desk.

A snake at least two-foot long began coiling its body around the man's wrist and struggling to wave its head. Its beady eyes stared at me. I was sure the thing was searching for the perfect place to bite.

So, you know, I did what I think most people would do in this situation: I jumped out of my chair and backwards, letting out a loud scream in the process. During this process, I tripped over the chair's rolling legs and started to fall back. My butt landed on the floor, but my head hit the seat of the chair, which I'm actually pretty thankful for, just because it would've been more mortifying to knock myself out, too.

Security saw some of this go down and came out to make sure I was okay, as if what happened wasn't embarrassing enough.

"It's just a little snake," one of the men said, as I bashfully refused his hand to get up off the floor.

That's sure not the way I saw it. When that thing looked in my direction, I think I entered the movie *Anaconda.*

"This thing bit my friend," the guy with the snake said. "His hand is already bruising and he says his heart has been racing since it happened. He can feel his blood clotting."

One of the security guys laughed. "It's just a rat snake. Your friend's gonna live, man."

I, on the other hand, was pretty sure I needed to check in for a heart attack.

Since I've started, I've seen more than a handful of patients who've been injured at a well-known store.

Most of the cases, I'd say, have been trivial. For example, if you fall in an aisle or a parking lot, or if **you** are pushing the cart and run your **own** toe over, it doesn't make a lot of sense to come in via ambulance six days later, screaming you're going to sue that business.

One case, I think I've seen, was serious enough to expect litigation.

In all cases, the patients have stated the business managers attempted to persuade them out of visiting the ER.

And in 9/10 cases, I wish they would've listened, instead of trying to build a case so they could become overnight millionaires.

Move-In Day at the Local College, Day Shift:

Patient was seen for an anxiety attack because she didn't realize this town didn't have a Starbucks or Target.

Staff concluded patient was falsifying claims to score medication and discharged her.

The Saddest Frequent Case

When I first started, I had patient come to the desk. She was a mute, so I guess it was no surprise to my coworker that the woman could not communicate when I asked her questions. My coworker handled the patient and later explained this elderly woman was a frequent flier. She would come with the complaint of urinary frequency.

Over time, I saw this patient at *least* 50 times. Sometimes I would see the woman three times a day. Times would pass when I would see the woman just once every other day. But no matter the frequency, we all knew her and were all concerned for her.

Clerks, security, doctors, and nurses expressed concern for this patient, and several of our staff members went to the point of calling social services. Repeatedly, the clerks on the other line told us they couldn't intervene; they gave us all a handful of excuses that didn't mean much to us because we were simply concerned about the patient's well-being, whereas they were concerned about the severity of the details we were presenting. I, for one, found it troubling that a 90-something-year-old could come in and tell us (write down) she couldn't remember that she had visited the ER three hours earlier than anything social services could tell us.

One night, the patient visited the ER department and was quickly discharged. She walked outside, and I didn't think much of it—until I just happened to glance up at the security monitors and saw the patient was wandering around our parking lot.

I left my desk and went outside.

"Do you need help?" I asked.

She nodded.

She pointed to a car, and then another, and then another, each time shrugging her shoulders. I came to the conclusion that the patient had forgotten where she'd parked. And, you know, that's no big deal, because I leave grocery stores sometimes and end up four rows away from my car.

We were outside for five minutes, walking all over the parking lot, before it hit me that something could be wrong.

I asked the patient to come inside with me, and we would help her find her car, but she refused. Doing the only thing I knew to do, I came inside and called security. I also informed the charge nurse of the unfolding events.

After 15 minutes of security helping the woman through the parking lot, they came to the realization that the woman had not driven to the hospital. She had ridden a bicycle, which was leaned up against the ER entrance.

The patient returned an hour later, with the same old chief complaint.

Social services was called at 2 a.m. and multiple staff members took over to insist upon an investigation.

Social services refused to participate, stating they could not intervene with a patient seeking healthcare.

The two ER doctors on shift called in a third and they all consulted and agreed to keep the patient in the ER. A mental health counselor was called, but concluded that the patient was of 'sound mind,' but only dealing with what she believed her life to be. The woman 'talked' all about her husband, about her family—she had three children and 18 grandkids.

Another call was made to social services when the patient returned for a third time in 24 hours.

This time, they stepped in and investigated.

According to social services, the patient's husband had passed some time ago, and the patient's children lived at least two hours away. It was only when the patient's husband had passed that she'd become a mute. She lost her voice the same time she lost her husband. But none of her children knew their mother had been struggling.

The patient was connected with her family, and her children made the joint decision to admit her to an assisted living facility.

Trust Your Family

We had a frequent flier—an elderly man—come in for generalized pain probably once a week. He was often given shots while in the hospital, and he was discharged with prescriptions for pain pills. He'd always show up with his son and daughter-in-law in tow, and he'd always leave with them. The two filled the man's prescriptions regularly.

After *months* of this man coming in, someone had the nerve to ask *why*. His answer was heartbreaking.

His son and daughter-in-law lived with him, and he was mostly okay with that, despite the two of them 'being messy' or 'having a circus of people over for company.' He needed help, and he said he felt his late wife would smack him upside the head if he turned away his only son, who'd been experiencing financial difficulties for some time, especially since the daughter-in-law was prone to what the old man called 'excessive' pregnancies and miscarriages when the man would finally break down and suggest the two find another place to live.

Well, the patient said he caught his son doing something wrong once. That 'something wrong' was the son emptying all the pain medication from the bottle to a bag, and then refilling the prescription bottle with OTC pain pills.

The elderly man refused to tell his story again to social services. Allegedly, he told the nurse he was afraid he would die alone, so he would live with the pain.

The nurse couldn't prove anything, and without the man's testimony, nothing could be done.

One night, I was working and I saw a discharge. The man had expired hours before I clocked in.

His son and daughter-in-law then became frequent fliers, checking in for any kind of pain you'd think possible.

"Do people always come in with sixteen family members or friends when they're here for headache?"-*My new coworker, as he observed the waiting room.*

My reply was, "Usually. And then they all get mad because only two visitors can go back at a time."

<u>Over and Over Again</u>

A man brought his sister in for abdominal pain, but he refused to go back to the room with her. That was no big deal.

So, the man took a seat in the waiting room and made himself comfortable by eating snacks from a bag he'd brought from home, drinking soda, and flipping through the TV channels by using an app on his phone that allowed him to use the device as a remote. He even rearranged furniture so he could prop his feet up on another chair and use one of the tables as a coffee table for his food and drink.

I thought this was clever. Nobody else was in the waiting room. He seemed okay, and that was great for me because I had tons of work to do. Again, no big deal.

Fifteen minutes after he and his sister had arrived, he came up to the desk and asked if he could have a blanket and a pillow. I was willing to give the man both, just because I knew I could do so without anyone else begging for the same. I went to the back for the items, and when I came back up to the desk, the man snatched the blanket and pillow from my hands without even the tiniest bit of gratitude.

"How long is this going to take?" he

demanded. He took long drinks from his coke bottle until he reached the center of the drink, and then he guzzled the rest down.

I tried to explain that patients presenting abdominal pain are usually in the ER for at least an hour.

Oh, the man threw a fit and wanted to know why. He wasn't satisfied when I then explained doctors and nurses need to order labs and such.

"Well, are they going to admit her?"

I glanced at the tracking board. By this time, the patient had been in the system for 22 minutes.

"I don't know," I told the man. "If you don't want to sit out here and wait, you're more than welcome to go back to her room. That way, you'll know a little more about what's going on."

The man furiously declined the offer and went back to the waiting room.

This happened four more times over the next hour, to the point that I was becoming just as angry as he was. Each time I offered to send him to his sister's room, he declined. I offered to get a nurse to come out and talk to him about what was going on. He declined.

The very last time the man came to the desk, I told him nothing had changed. I still had no information I could give him about how much longer it would be, didn't know if his sister would be admitted, and added that it had been a busy shift before he and his sister arrived, so we all had a lot of work to catch up on. I explained more than half of our rooms were occupied and they were short two nurses in the back. I tried to be as nice as possible when trying to get him to understand that I had other things to do than continue to go through this time and time again.

"Well, if you only have half of the rooms used, that means the other half are empty. You guys aren't that busy. You're just lazy."

I went to find the charge nurse and explained I had hit my limit with the patient's brother. She was buried in paperwork and all of the nurses in back were struggling to catch up on charting. She said she'd come up to talk to the man, so I headed back up front. On the way up there, I noticed the man's sister was doubled over in her bed.

"A nurse is coming up to speak with you," I told the patient's brother.

He flew off the handle.

"I didn't ask for that. I didn't ask you to get anyone else involved."

I shook my head. "I can't answer any of your questions, so I found someone to help."

A few minutes later, the charge nurse emerged from the back. By this time, the patient's brother had returned to the waiting room and was laughing at something on TV.

"Sir," the charge nurse said, "I hear you were asking about your sister, and I may be able to help you out a little."

"What?" he asked, with an innocent expression. "I haven't left his waiting room one time. Just watchin' my shows and waiting for you fine professionals to do what you need to do."

I gritted my teeth.

The charge nurse wasn't going to argue with him, so she instead just informed the man they were still unsure of how long his sister would be in the ER, didn't know yet if she would be admitted, and talked to him about the first few test results they'd seen.

He thanked her and she returned to the back. No sooner than she disappeared through the triage door, the brother was at the desk again.

"You're kidding me, right?" I asked him.

I guess the charge nurse believed me when I told her the man was causing trouble, because she never went to the back. She walked through triage and waited in the hallway so she could hear when the man came back up.

The second he started yelling at me, the charge nurse stomped out to the lobby and informed the man of his two options: sit down and shut up, or leave.

He agreed to sit down.

"Wait," the charge nurse said, as the man passed closely by her. "You smell like alcohol. Are you drinking while you're in my waiting room?"

BINGO!

The patient's brother had poured Jack Daniels in a few bottles of coke before leaving home.

His sister was admitted for pancreatitis. He

was escorted off hospital property by two fine police officers because he became belligerent when security told him he needed to find a ride home.

The triage nurse was reading the newspaper one night and came across an article that featured one of our frequent drug seekers.

The man was arrested for harming his dog so he could take the pet's pain pills.

I want to say 'Only in Ohio,' but I'm pretty sure this is becoming increasingly popular elsewhere as well.

Evening shift, time unknown, tracking board full.

A male college kid presented for bumps on his penis.

He waited in the waiting room for two hours before he was taken back to a non-trauma room for examination.

Doctor diagnosed him with genital herpes.

Patient hit on literally every female staff member he encountered.

He left without a date.

Things I Frequently Hear from the Triage Room:

-I didn't bring my med list, but it should all be in your system.

-I don't know what the pill is called. It's blue, though.

-But her fever was 103 at home. It just *can't* be 97.4 right now. We only left three minutes ago.

-Nothing's changed except [I no longer take 10/12 medications listed, I am divorced, was diagnosed with three major illnesses, and I'm pregnant], so I don't know why you have to ask me all these questions.

-My pain is a 10/10. "So what's the highest pain you can tolerate?" Patient: A 10. "But you're not handling this very well, or you wouldn't be here, so what can we get it down to?" Patient: A zero.

-Do you think I'm going to be admitted?

-You mean I have to go *back* to the waiting

room? I've already been waiting 20 minutes.

-My doctor said he called and told you all of this already.

- "Well..." *This is how you know you're about to hear the patient's entire life story.*

-I've had this pain for thirty years, but tonight is the night you're going to make it go away.

-Can I go out for a smoke before you take me back?

-When the triage nurse asks when the pain/symptoms started, some patients reply, "After I got off work." Okay...Yesterday? Today? At 1? At 7?

-Oh, I didn't know it still counted that I have high blood pressure/diabetes/heart problems if I am taking pills for it.

-Dog dander, apple-scented lotion, those pine tree air fresheners, papaya, a plant native to Maui that doesn't grow around here, red dye #34, not allergic to the sun but I burn really bad when I'm in it, poison ivy, poison sumac, got bit by a spider once and my arm swelled up so spiders, mosquitoes do the same thing come to think of it, and pineapple. *Patients, when asked if they are allergic to anything.*

In case you were wondering, yes, we have patients who whip out photo IDs and insurance cards from bras, underwear, and socks...

Secret Garden

A 16-ish-year-old-girl was brought to the desk by her mother for a complaint of abdominal pain.

I was able to register the patient quickly and the bedside registration was going smoothly, until the nurse came in and told the patient it was shot time. This shot was going to be administered to her upper hip/buttocks region, so the patient was told she was going to need to open her gown a little.

Well, this is when the girl started freaking out. She didn't seem a bit upset that she was going to get a shot, but she sure was panicking over *where* she was getting it.

I thanked the girl's mother for answering my questions, wished the patient good luck, and I left the room with my cart so that I could finish the patient's chart in the hallway.

Now, some of our patients seem to think nobody else can hear what's going on in a specific room, just because there's a curtain there for 'privacy.' Maybe some don't really care, I don't know. With this girl, I'm thinking it was the latter.

"You're not giving me a shot in my butt. Can't you give it in my arm or something?"

"Just open your gown a little and get it over

with," mom scolded.

"But can't it be in my arm? Or thigh? Or anywhere but here?"

The nurse tried to coax the girl. At one point, I think the teen was sobbing.

Finally, mom said, "We can go get people to help hold you down, if you can't act right and just let her stick you."

I guess the girl calmed down and opened her gown.

"Jane Allison Doe!" mom shrieked.

Honestly, I was thinking the patient tried to bite the nurse or something. I couldn't think of anything else that would warrant that kind of scathing, surprised response from the teen's mother.

"It's just a little flower, mom," the teen explained.

"That's not *just* a flower, Jane. You have a garden tattooed across your ass."

Well, that sure answered my question of 'What is going on in there?'

Mom immediately swooped in and wanted to know when her daughter had the artwork done, and then shifted focus to the fact that the girl had to have been partially nude when receiving the tattoo that ran from the small of her back, over both buttocks, and partially down her hips (I was able to gather this from the argument and the nurse's testimony).

I went back to the front and could occasionally

hear the two shouting at each other. They were still fighting when they left the ER.

Wow.

I was hanging out in the back hallway, finishing up a chart, when a trauma patient coded. As to be expected, most of the nurses and doctors in the department sprinted to the man's room and began trying to save his life.

This didn't surprise me, and neither did other patients peeking out of their rooms or actually leaving their rooms to stand in the hall and try to see the action. That kind of stuff actually happens a lot more than people think.

What completely floored me, however, was the mother of one of our non-critical frequent fliers, this time in for something like a sore throat. She watched as staff members were frantically pushing meds and doing CPR, but it was as if she couldn't care less. She walked right up to the coding patient's room, approached a nurse, and stated her son needed a warm blanket.

I still love my job, even on the days I'm just
barely hanging on!

Made in the USA
San Bernardino, CA
03 October 2018